Communication Skills in Pharmacy Practice

A Practical Guide for Students and Practitioners

SIXTH EDITION

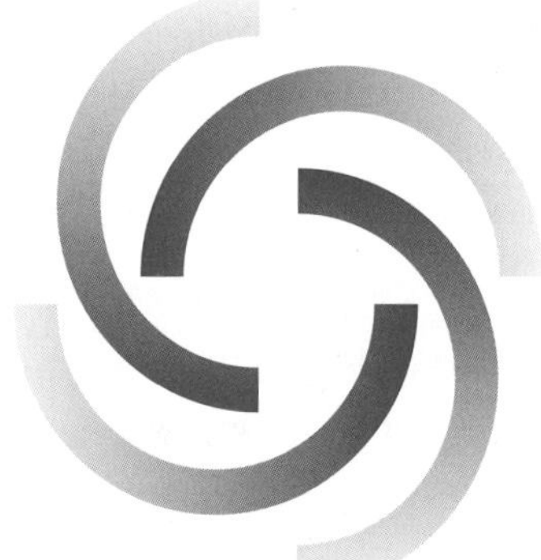

Wolters Kluwer | Lippincott Williams & Wilkins
Health

Philadelphia • Baltimore • New York • London
Buenos Aires • Hong Kong • Sydney • Tokyo

Acquisitions Editor: David Troy
Product Manager: Matt Hauber
Marketing Manager: Allison Powell
Designer: Steve Druding
Production Service: SPi Global

Two Commerce Square
2001 Market Street
Philadelphia, PA 19103
LWW.com

Printed in China.

Library of Congress Cataloging-in-Publication Data

Communication skills in pharmacy practice : a practical guide for students and practitioners / [edited by] Robert S. Beardsley, Carole L. Kimberlin, William N. Tindall. — 6th ed.

p. ; cm.

Includes bibliographical references and index.

ISBN 978-1-60831-602-1

1. Communication in pharmacy. 2. Pharmacist and patient. I. Beardsley, Robert S. II. Kimberlin, Carole L. III. Tindall, William N.

[DNLM: 1. Communication. 2. Pharmacists. 3. Professional-Patient Relations. QV 21]

RS56.C65 2013

615′.1—dc23

2011023987

To purchase additional copies of this book, call our customer service department at (800) 638-3030 or fax orders to (301) 223-232 0. International customers should call (301) 223-2300.
Visit Lippincott Williams & Wilkins on the Internet at LWW.com. Lippincott Williams & Wilkins customer service representatives are available from 8:30 am to 6 pm, EST.

10 9 8 7 6 5 4 3 2 1

CCS1111

Communication Skills in Pharmacy Practice

A Practical Guide for Students and Practitioners

SIXTH EDITION

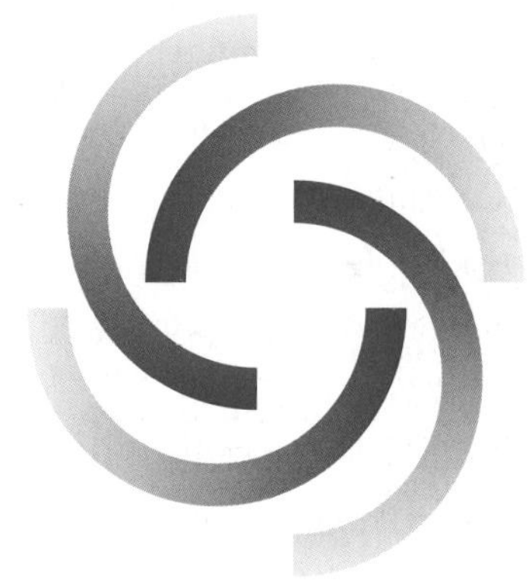

Robert S. Beardsley, PhD, RPh

Professor

Department of Pharmaceutical Health Services Research

University of Maryland School of Pharmacy

Baltimore, Maryland

Carole L. Kimberlin, PhD

Professor

Department of Pharmacy Health Care Administration

University of Florida College of Pharmacy

Gainesville, Florida

William N. Tindall, PhD, RPh

Professor Emeritus

Department of Family Medicine

Alliance for Research in Community Health

Wright State University School of Medicine

Dayton, Ohio

To Kathy, Kyle, and Jessica; Philip;
Sylvia, Christine, Laura, Michael, and Aidan
for Communicating the Lessons of Love

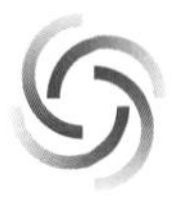

Contributors

Chapter 11

Betsy L. Sleath, PhD
Chair and Professor of Pharmaceutical Outcomes and Policy
University of North Carolina Eshelman School of Pharmacy
Chapel Hill, North Carolina

Patricia J. Bush, PhD
Professor Emeritus
Georgetown University School of Medicine
Washington, District of Columbia

Chapter 13

Jeff J. Cain, EdD
Director of Education Technology and Adjunct Associate Professor
University of Kentucky College of Pharmacy
Lexington, Kentucky

Kevin A. Clauson, PharmD
Associate Professor
Nova Southeastern University College of Pharmacy
Fort Lauderdale, Florida

Brent I. Fox, PharmD, PhD
Assistant Professor
Auburn University - Harrison School of Pharmacy
Auburn, Alabama

Chapter 14

Mona M. Sedrak, PhD, PA-C
Physician Assistant Program Chair and Associate Professor
Seton Hall University, School of Health and Medical Sciences
South Orange, New Jersey

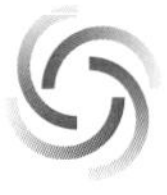

Preface

Interpersonal communication is the foundation of patient-centered care. Without clear communication, desired patient outcomes cannot be achieved. Unclear messages between pharmacy personnel and other health care providers lead to errors in medication therapy management. Failed communication between pharmacy staff and patients promotes unsafe medication use. Pharmacists have a responsibility to not only dispense appropriate medications but also to ensure patient understanding of the medications they use. Pharmacists and their staffs must acknowledge the value of interpersonal communication as an essential element in building trust between patients and the pharmacy community. Interpersonal communication often appears to be a simple process at first glance; however, as revealed in this textbook, interpersonal skill development is a complex process requiring a lifelong commitment to improvement and practice.

What is New in this Edition

In this sixth edition, you will find new principles, practices, and procedures that will contribute to your ability to promote good health outcomes for patients. Communication has become even more important as health care continues to evolve at a quickening pace. Health care in general and pharmacy in particular have undergone dramatic changes in recent years that have affected pharmacists' professional roles and responsibilities. For example, state pharmacy statutes and regulations now include new definitions of the scope of pharmacy practice that involve the concepts of medication therapy management. Another example is the opportunity for new services and compensation offered under the coding schemes of Medicare Part D. A third example is the increasing role of pharmacists in public health. One final example is the heightened public awareness of daily tragedies in which people become ill and even die as a result of improper prescribing and inappropriate use of medication.

Health care is undergoing a shift to more patient-centered models of care in which patients are actively involved in making decisions about treatments, setting goals for treatment, and monitoring outcomes of care. As pharmacists and their staffs participate in more patient-centered care, they must strengthen their interpersonal communication skills. As discussed in this textbook, evidence is accumulating that patient outcomes are enhanced by providers who communicate more effectively and build more positive relationships with the patients they serve.

To reflect this evolution in health care, all the chapters have been substantially updated and revised for this edition. Furthermore, contemporary issues continue to be added to several chapters, including Chapter 8, "Helping Patients Manage

Therapeutic Regimens"; Chapter 9, "Medication Safety and Communication Skills"; Chapter 12, "Communication Skills and Interprofessional Collaboration"; and Chapter 13, "Electronic Communication in Health Care."

Organizational Philosophy

Each chapter builds on the one preceding it. This book first focuses on defining interpersonal communication and its various components. The initial chapters help you better understand communication, which can be a fragile process, and appreciate the importance of effective communication to your success in pharmacy:

- Chapter 1 describes the characteristics of patient-centered pharmaceutical care.
- Chapter 2 provides an interactive model of interpersonal communication that can help you analyze and understand the communication process.
- Chapters 3 and 4 identify crucial nonverbal elements in communication and examine environmental and personal barriers to effective communication with patients that must be addressed in pharmacy practice.
- Chapter 5 focuses on the crucial roles that effective listening and empathic communication play in your ability to establish effective, trusting relationships with the patients you serve.
- Chapter 6 identifies aspects of assertiveness that will help you both initiate effective communication and respond appropriately in conflict situations with patients, coworkers, physicians, and other health care professionals.

In the remaining chapters, we provide specific strategies on using these skills in a variety of practice situations:

- Chapter 7 presents the most common approaches to interviewing patients and assessing their needs. The effective collection and organizing of patient data is built on strong listening, interviewing, and assessment skills. It is difficult to provide patient-centered care without clear and comprehensive information.
- Chapter 8, which builds on these interviewing and assessment skills, presents the most appropriate strategies for helping patients with medication management issues. Relevant areas of discovery that influence your strategies include understanding the reasons why patients may not take medications correctly and how patient outcomes can be enhanced using effective communication skills. Motivational Interviewing is discussed as a possible strategy.
- Chapter 9 continues the discussion about how effective interpersonal communication enhances patient care and describes the role of communication in minimizing medication errors and improving patient safety. The evidence is rather stunning about the frequency and seriousness of errors due to lack of effective communication.
- Chapter 10 demonstrates that application of these skills to specific patient populations is essential since different approaches and sensitivities are needed for various types of patients. The key is to be aware of the general

characteristics of specific populations and their unique needs without stereotyping individuals or making invalid assumptions. The chapter illustrates the fact that the more you know about your patient, the more effective you will be in developing a targeted strategy to assist them with medication adherence.

- Chapter 11 covers strategies for interacting with children and their families, since this population requires unique approaches.
- Chapter 12 provides insights into interprofessional communication and the development of critical collaborative relationships with other health care providers in an effort to enhance patient care. Developing these relationships requires many of the communication skills described in earlier chapters. This chapter serves as an excellent illustration of how communication skills are put into action, especially in light of the increased emphasis on interprofessional education.
- Chapter 13 identifies communication skills that are essential to assuring patient safety and better health care outcomes using e-communication. Due to advances in technology, more and more communication is being conducted electronically rather than person-to-person; therefore, pharmacists and pharmacy technicians need to learn how communication skills apply to this medium.
- The final chapter, Chapter 14, frames pharmacy interactions with others in the broader context of appropriate and inappropriate behavior. Experience has shown that how and why pharmacists and their staffs interact with others (as viewed from an ethical framework) influences their effectiveness in working with patients and other health care providers.

Pedagogical Features of the Book

Communication Skills in Pharmacy Practice, Sixth Edition, contains the following elements geared toward enhancing learning and improving communication skills:

- Chapter overview: This section serves as an introductory text to inform the reader what topics will be covered in the chapter.
- Case studies: These example scenarios, many based on actual situations, involve practical application of communication skills. Many of the case studies include dialogue and analysis that illustrate skills discussed in the text.
- Boxes: Important concepts are highlighted in boxes throughout the text. These nuggets summarize information or provide examples that complement chapter discussions.
- Summary: Each chapter ends with a summary underscoring the chapter's main points, ensuring that the reader retains the most important knowledge presented.
- Review questions and review cases: Review problems reinforce concepts learned in the chapter. Answers to these questions or cases are available to the instructor (see the "Instructor's Manuals" section below).
- References and suggested readings: The final element of each chapter is a list of references cited in the text. Some chapters include sources that we suggest readers review for additional information.

Strategies for Improving Communication

Throughout the text, we describe strategies to improve communication skills. Improvement implies that behaviors that inhibit communication must be altered. The interpersonal communication skills described in this book are learned skills, which take practice to master. Many pharmacists and their staffs have not practiced these skills to the point they are comfortable applying them. The net result is that they either avoid uncomfortable situations or they hesitate or "freeze" when confronted with a new situation. When attempting to change communication behaviors, it is important for you to think about your own goals for improvement and to develop strategies to deal with needed changes.

As a guide, the following sequence of activities has been shown to be effective in modifying communication behaviors:

1. Being aware of the various communication elements (what these elements are, which ones are the most important, how you use them, which approach is the best)
2. Practicing these skills (actually using these strategies in interactions)
3. Assessing the approach (what went well, what needs to be improved)

Following this assessment, a new sequence should follow:

1. Awareness (what should be done differently next time)
2. Practice (conducting the new strategy)
3. Assessment (whether it worked this time, what could be done differently next time)

Many times, this sequence needs to be followed by another cycle (awareness, practice, assessment, and so on) until you feel you have met your goals. Hopefully, you will appreciate the fact that communication skill development is an ongoing learning process. We hope you enjoy the journey of learning about this important area and developing these skills.

Additional Resources

For faculty adopting the book, two instructor's manuals—one geared toward instructors of pharmacy students and one geared toward instructors of pharmacy technician students—can be accessed at http://thePoint.lww.com/beardsley6e.

At the same Web site, students can access videos demonstrating the effective use of communication skills and strategies.

ACKNOWLEDGMENTS

The editors would like to thank several individuals for their contributions to this edition. True appreciation goes first to faculty members who have used this textbook throughout the years and have provided us with valuable feedback about its utility and effectiveness, and next, to the students and to the practicing pharmacists and their staffs who have enhanced their communication skill development using this book and who must learn how to communicate with patients, their families, and other health care providers in today's challenging pharmacy practice environment.

We appreciate the assistance of our contributing authors in shaping the message and application of material in the textbook—we certainly appreciate your insights. We also acknowledge the assistance of the following individuals in the various photographs used in the book: Jennifer Huang, Brian Hose, Meredith Brittain, and Carrie Filsinger. In addition, we are grateful to Sean Parsons, B.S., CPhT, a pharmacy instructor at Bidwell Training Center, Inc., who created the pharmacy technician instructor's manual for the book.

Robert S. Beardsley
Baltimore, Maryland

Carole L. Kimberlin
Gainesville, Florida

William N. Tindall
Chesterfield, Virginia

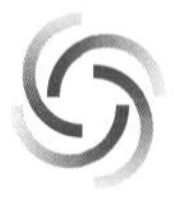

Contents

CHAPTER

1

Patient-Centered Communication in Pharmacy Practice

Overview

In order to meet their professional responsibilities, pharmacists have become more patient-centered in their provision of pharmaceutical care. Pharmacists have the potential to contribute even more to improved patient care through efforts to reduce medication errors and improve the use of medications by patients. Using effective communication skills is essential in the provision of patient care. This chapter describes key elements within patient-centered care and introduces the critical nature of communication to this process. Subsequent chapters provide specific examples of communication skill development and strategies to enhance patient-centered communication.

Introduction

Why is patient-centered communication so crucial to a professional practice? Consider the following:

- A 36-year-old man was prescribed a fentanyl patch to treat pain resulting from a back injury. He was not informed that heat could make the patch unsafe to use.

He fell asleep with a heating pad and died. The level of fentanyl in his bloodstream was found to be 100 times the level it should have been (Fallik, 2006).

- A patient prescribed Normodyne for hypertension (HTN) was dispensed Norpramin. She experienced numerous side effects, including blurred vision and hand tremors. Since she knew that she was supposed to be taking the medication to treat HTN, even minimal communication between the pharmacist and patient about the therapy would have prevented this medication error (ISMP, 2004).
- An 83-year-old patient was given Cardizem CD (sustained-release diltiazem capsules) for blood pressure control. Because the capsule was too large to swallow, the patient chewed the medication. As a result, her pulse slowed twice to low levels, and the family contacted the pharmacist for advice. Upon learning that she was chewing the medication, the pharmacist suggested that the physician substitute immediate-release diltiazem tablets, which are easier to swallow. The prescription was changed and the patient did well for several months. Months later, the patient returned to her physician for a checkup. She was again put on Cardizem CD. She again began chewing the larger capsules. She became progressively weaker and died 3 weeks later (ISMP, 2010).
- A study by Weingart et al. (2005) found that, while 27% of patients experienced symptoms they attributed to a new prescription, many of these symptoms (31%) were not reported to the prescribing physician. The first author reported in a news release that "For every symptom that patients experienced but failed to report, one in five resulted in an adverse drug event that could have been prevented or made less severe." Authors' speculation on why patients failed to report symptoms focused on health care providers who do not inquire about problems with drug therapy and patients who dismiss the seriousness of side effects or do not want to be seen as complaining to physicians about treatments prescribed for them.

Pharmacists are accepting increased responsibility in assuring that patients avoid adverse effects of medications and reach desired outcomes from their therapies. The changing role of the pharmacist requires practitioners to switch from a "medication-centered" or "task-centered" practice to patient-centered care. As revealed in the situations described above, it is not enough for pharmacists and their staffs to simply provide medication in the most efficient and safest manner (i.e., focus on systems of drug order fulfillment). Pharmacists must participate in activities that enhance patient adherence and the wise use of medication (i.e., focus on patient-centered elements including patient understanding and actual medication-taking behaviors). Patient-centered care depends on your ability to develop trusting relationships with patients, to engage in an open exchange of information, to involve patients in the decision-making process regarding treatment, and to help patients reach therapeutic goals that are understood and endorsed by patients as well as by health care providers. Effective communication is central to meeting these patient care responsibilities in the practice of pharmacy.

Pharmacists' Responsibility in Patient Care

The incidence of preventable adverse drug events and the cost to society associated with medication-related morbidity and mortality are of growing concern (Ernst and Grizzle, 2001; Gurwitz et al., 2003; Rodriguez-Monguio et al., 2003; Easton et al., 2004; Field et al., 2005 ; Krähenbühl-Melcher et al., 2007; Rogers, 2009).

The Institute of Medicine (IOM) report on patient safety concluded that medication-related errors are among the most prevalent errors in medical care (Committee on Quality of Health Care in America, 1999). The potential of pharmacists to play a pivotal role in reducing the incidence of both medication-related errors and drug-related illness is also receiving increased attention (Hepler and Strand, 1990; Leape et al., 1999; Hepler, 2001; Cranor et al., 2003; Bunting and Cranor, 2006; Schnipper et al., 2006; Pai, 2009; Westerlund and Marklund, 2009).

Hepler and Strand (1990) have made a compelling case for the societal need for pharmaceutical care, which they define as "the responsible provision of drug therapy for the purpose of achieving definite outcomes that improve a patient's quality of life." Reports from the Council on Credentialing for Pharmacy, "*Scope of Contemporary Pharmacy Practice: Roles, Responsibilities, and Functions of Pharmacists and Pharmacy Technicians*" (Council on Credentialing for Pharmacy, 2009) and the Joint Commission of Pharmacy Practitioners, "*Future Vision of Pharmacy Practice*" (Joint Commission of Pharmacy Practitioners, 2008), highlight pharmacist roles in this important area. Mission statements of professional pharmacy associations have been changed in recent years to reflect the increased responsibility pharmacists are being asked to assume for the appropriate use of drugs in society.

The "patient-centered" role envisioned by pharmacy mission statements would afford pharmacists a value to society far beyond that provided by their "drug-centered" role. However, while the mission statements of professional organizations can help guide practice, they must be translated into patient care activities that pharmacists provide to each of their patients. The quality of the interpersonal relationships pharmacists develop with patients depends upon effective communication.

Importance of Communication in Meeting Your Patient Care Responsibilities

The communication process between you and your patients serves two primary functions:

1. It establishes the ongoing relationship between you and your patients.
2. It provides the exchange of information necessary to assess your patients' health conditions, reach decisions on treatment plans, implement the plans, and evaluate the effects of treatment on your patients' quality of life.

Establishing trusting relationships with your patients is not simply something that is "nice to do" but is essential to the "real" purpose of pharmacy practice. The quality of the patient–provider relationship is crucial. All professional activities between you and your patients take place in the context of the relationship that you establish. An effective relationship forms the base that allows you to meet professional responsibilities in patient care.

The ultimate purpose of the professional–patient relationship must constantly be kept in mind. The purpose of the relationship is to achieve mutually understood and agreed upon goals for therapy that improve your patients' quality of life. Your activities must, therefore, be thought of in terms of the patient outcomes that you help reach. You must begin to redefine what you do with the focus being on patient needs. Your goal, for example, is changed from providing patients with drug information to a goal of assuring that patients understand their treatment in order to take medications safely and appropriately. Your goal is not to get patients to do as they are told (i.e., comply) but to help them reach intended treatment outcomes. Providing information or trying to improve adherence must each be seen as a means to reaching a desired outcome rather than being an end in itself. Even communication with your patients is not an end in itself. Conversation between you and your patient has a different purpose than conversation between friends. Patient–professional communication is a means to an end—that of establishing a therapeutic relationship in order to effectively provide health care services that the patient needs. Patient well-being is paramount. Because of your unique knowledge and special societal responsibilities, you must bear the greater burden of assuring effective communication in your patient encounters.

What is Patient-Centered Care?

Mead and Bower (2000) describe five dimensions of patient-centered medical care (see Box 1.1) that help shape the following discussion. Models of the

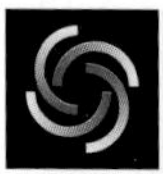

BOX 1.1 Providing Patient-Centered Care

The pharmacist must be able to:

- Understand all aspects of the patient's illness experience: the social, psychological, and biomedical factors
- Perceive each patient as a person; understand the patient's unique experience of illness and the "personal meaning" it entails
- Foster a more egalitarian relationship with patients; allow patients to be actively involved in dialogue and in the decision-making surrounding treatment
- Build a "therapeutic alliance" with patients by incorporating patient perceptions of the acceptability of interventions in treatment plans, defining mutually agreed-upon goals for treatment, and establishing a trusting, caring relationship with the patient
- Develop self-awareness of his or her personal effects on patients and how his or her own responses to patients may affect patient behavior

prescribing process that are "practitioner-centered" have primarily focused on decisions made and actions taken by physicians and other health care providers. The patient is "acted upon" rather than being viewed as an active participant who makes ongoing decisions affecting the outcomes of treatment. The patient is seen as the object of professional ministrations and as the cooperative (or recalcitrant) follower of professional dictates.

One of our professional conceits seems to be that prescribing and dispensing a medication are the key decisions in the medication use process. However, in most cases, it is the patient who must return home and carry out the prescribed treatment. The traditional model of health care focused on provision of acute, institutionalized care. However, chronic disease care consumes approximately 75% of health care resources (Centers for Disease Control and Prevention, 2009). Drug therapy is the most ubiquitous of medical interventions and, in ambulatory care, is largely managed by the patient. The degree of autonomy that is possible with medication therapy makes it likely that patients will make decisions and assert control over treatment in various ways. Many patients make autonomous decisions to alter treatment regimens—decisions that may be made without consultation or communication with you or other health care providers (Heath et al., 2002; Wroe, 2002; George et al., 2005; Lowry et al., 2005; Pound et al., 2005). Ignorance of patient-initiated decisions on medication use, in turn, makes it difficult for health care professionals to accurately evaluate the effects of drug treatment.

While you may view such patient behavior as ill-advised, it would be more helpful for you to acknowledge the fact that patients do exercise ultimate control over drug treatment. Rather than trying to stifle patient autonomy, it would be more productive to strengthen the therapeutic alliance with your patients by increasing the level of patient participation and control in decisions that are made about treatment. Patient perceptions that you "care" for them (as well as providing care) are essential to the establishment of trust. Examination of reasons for filing malpractice claims against providers suggests that patient anger over a perceived lack of "caring" from providers and dissatisfaction with provider communication were important elements in decisions to file (Hickson et al., 1992; Spector, 2010).

Encouraging a More Active Patient Role in Therapeutic Monitoring

Providers, including pharmacists, could do more to help enable patients and their family or caregivers to take a more active role in monitoring response to treatment. The information a patient provides you as part of therapeutic monitoring is essential to assuring that treatment goals are being met. While INR or HbA1c values may provide the comfort of a "scientific" basis for therapeutic monitoring, for many chronic conditions you must rely on patient report of response to treatment. Treatment of depression and pain, for example, have only patient self-report as the basis of evaluation of response to therapy. Many other conditions such as asthma, angina, GERD, epilepsy, and arthritis rely heavily on patient report of symptoms.

In addition to conditions where patient report of symptomatic experience is critical to monitoring, research has documented the beneficial effects on patient outcomes of increased patient involvement in self-monitoring of physiological indicators of treatment effectiveness. Certainly, patient self-monitoring of blood glucose has become standard practice in managing diabetes. In addition, blood glucose awareness training (BGAT) programs teach patients to recognize signs of both hyperglycemia and hypoglycemia. The BGAT programs have been found to improve a patient's ability to accurately estimate blood glucose fluctuations and prevent severe hypoglycemic episodes (Cox et al., 1994, 2001; Schachinger et al., 2005). Programs to increase patient participation in monitoring of coagulation therapy along with protocol-based patient management of warfarin dosing have led to reduced incidence of major bleeding in patient monitoring intervention groups (Beyth et al., 2000; Ryan et al., 2009).

The Veterans Health Administration implemented a national home telehealth program to provide routine chronic care management services for diabetes mellitus, congestive heart failure, HTN, posttraumatic stress disorder, chronic obstructive pulmonary disease, and depression, with monitoring data transmitted electronically (Darkins et al., 2008). Biometric devices monitor vital signs. Videotelemonitors are used to conduct consultations in the home in place of in-person examinations. These initiatives point to the sophistication with which patients can monitor response to therapy and make informed decisions when they are taught how to interpret both symptomatic experience and results of physiological tests.

Other programs have designed interventions to teach patients how to be more assertive in obtaining information from providers. Intervention group subjects were found to be more likely than control subjects to question providers (Roter, 1984; Greenfield et al., 1985, 1988; Kaplan et al., 1989; Kimberlin et al., 2001) following the training intervention. In addition, patient follow-up found that intervention group patients had improved health outcomes, including improved glycemic control in diabetic patients, up to a year following the interventions (Greenfield et al., 1985; Kaplan et al., 1989).

The Joint Commission and the Agency for Healthcare Research and Quality (AHRQ) have published tips for patients to empower them to be more active in their own treatment and in decisions made on their care (AHRQ, 2002; Joint Commission, 2002; NCPIE, 2006). As an example, one tip for surgery patients from The Joint Commission states: "Don't be afraid to ask about safety. If you're having surgery, for example, ask the physician to mark the area that is to be operated upon, so that there's no confusion in the operating room." Other pieces of advice include: "Make sure you can read the handwriting on any prescriptions written by your doctor. If you can't read it, the pharmacist may not be able to either," and "If you are given an IV, ask the nurse how long it should take for the liquid to 'run out.' Tell the nurse if it doesn't seem to be dripping properly (that it is too fast or too slow)." While this advice is important in promoting more patient-centered care, patients must be taught how to be more involved in decision making. In addition, their assertiveness must be encouraged and reinforced by all health care providers involved in their care in order for such a dramatic change from the traditional role of the patient to be embraced. If some providers, in fact, punish the patient for asking more questions and being more assertive, your attempts to establish more patient-centered care could be undone.

A Patient-Centered View of the Medication Use Process

A patient-centered view of the medication use process focuses on the patient role in the process. The medication use process for noninstitutionalized patients begins when the patient perceives a health care need or health-related problem. This is experienced as a deviation from what is "normal" for the individual. It may be the experience of "symptoms" or another sort of lifestyle interruption that challenges or threatens the patient's sense of well-being. The patient then interprets the perceived problem. This interpretation is influenced by a host of psychological and social factors unique to the individual. These include the individual's previous experience with the formal health care system; family influences; cultural differences in the conceptualization of "health" and "illness"; knowledge of the problem (individuals vary greatly in levels of medical and biological knowledge); health beliefs that may or may not coincide with accepted medical "truths"; psychological characteristics; personal values, motives, and goals; and so on. In addition, the patient's interpretation may be influenced by outside forces, such as family members who offer their own interpretations and advice.

The patient at this point may take no action to treat the condition, either because the problem is seen as minor or transitory or because the patient lacks the means to initiate treatment. If the patient takes action, the action can include initiation of self-treatment, initiation of contact with a nonmedical provider (such as a faith healer), and/or contact with a health care provider. If the patient takes action that involves contact with a health care professional, whether it be physician, pharmacist, or other health care practitioner, he must describe his "symptom" experience and to some extent his interpretation of that experience. In many ways, it is at this point that control gets transferred from the patient to the professional, for it is the professional who can legitimize the experience by giving it a name (diagnosis). Such an act, however, transforms the experience from that with patient meaning into that with practitioner meaning (which may or may not be shared by the patient). The quality of the professional assessment depends, in part, on the thoroughness of the patient report, the practitioner's skill in eliciting relevant information, and the receptivity of the professional to "hear" information from the patient that is potentially important. The practitioner's skill in communicating information about the diagnosis may alter or refine the patient's conceptualization of his or her illness experience, making patient understanding more congruent with that of the health care provider.

Once the health care providers reach a professional assessment or diagnosis of the patient's problem based on patient report, patient examination, and other data, they make a recommendation to the patient. If the recommendation is to initiate medication treatment, patients may or may not carry out the recommendation. Data indicate that large numbers of prescriptions are written that are never filled (Safran et al., 2005; Olson et al., 2005) or are filled but remain unclaimed in the pharmacy (Kinnaird et al., 2003). Approximately 20% of people report that they take less prescription medication than recommended because of cost (Reed and Hargraves, 2003; Piette et al., 2004, 2006; Soumerai et al., 2006). Failure to initiate prescribed therapy may be caused by economic constraints, a lack of understanding of the purpose of the recommendation, or failure to "buy into" the treatment plan. Some of these patient decisions may, in fact, reflect a failure in the communication process between the patient and the health care provider.

When patients do accept the recommendations to initiate drug treatment, obtain the medication, and attempt to follow the regimen as prescribed, they can do so only to the best of their ability as they understand the drugs are intended to be taken. For many patients, medication taking includes misuse caused by misunderstanding of what is recommended or by unintended deviations from the prescribed treatment regimen (e.g., doses are forgotten). Alternatively, patients may administer the medication but with intentional modifications of the regimen. In both unintentional and intentional modifications of the prescribed treatment, the patient's actions may be influenced by how well you and other health care providers succeed in establishing mutually understood and agreed-upon treatment plans. Regardless of the medication-taking practices that patients establish, they evaluate the consequences of the treatment in terms of perceived benefits and perceived costs or barriers. This evaluation results in patients continuing to take the medications, patients altering their drug treatment regimens, or patients discontinuing drug therapy.

In any case, patients are continuously estimating what they perceive the effects of their actions to be and adjusting their behavior accordingly. It is inevitable that, as patients begin medication treatment, they will "monitor" their own response—they will decide whether or not they feel differently; they will look for signs that the treatment is effective or, alternately, indications that there may be a problem with the medication. The problem is not that patients monitor their response to medications—it is inevitable and desirable that they do so. The problem that exists is that patients often lack information on what to expect from treatment—on what to look for that will give them valid feedback on their response to the medication. Lacking this information, they apply their own "common sense" criteria.

When possible, you should encourage patients to share their experience with therapy (see Box 1.2). Patients may interrupt the treatment process by failing to contact you and other providers when follow-up is expected, which may involve discontinuing participation in the formal health care system for a period of time or contacting a new provider and beginning the whole process again. Of the patients who do contact their providers, some will communicate their

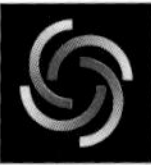

BOX 1.2 Pharmacists Should Encourage Patients to Share Their Experiences With Therapy

- They may have unanswered questions.
- They may have misunderstandings or misperceptions.
- They may experience problems related to therapy and not tell you.
- They may "monitor" their own response to treatment without involving you.
- They may make their own decisions regarding therapy.
- They may not reveal key information to you unless you initiate a dialogue.

perceptions, problems, and decisions regarding treatment. Other patients may contact providers and *not* convey this information (or not convey all pertinent aspects). This follow-up contact occurs during revisits with a physician or refills of prescriptions from pharmacists. The nature of their relationships with you and other providers, the degree to which patients feel "safe" in confiding difficulties or concerns, the skill of providers in eliciting patient perceptions, and the extent to which a sense of "partnership" has been established regarding treatment decisions all influence the patient decision to recontact providers. These factors also influence the degree to which medication-taking practices are reported and perceptions shared. Regardless of how completely patients report their experience with therapy when they recontact providers, the provider will make a professional assessment of patient response to treatment based on what the patient does report and/or lab values and other physiological measures. This assessment will lead to recommendations to continue drug treatment as previously recommended, to alter drug treatment (i.e., to change dose, change drug, add drug), or to discontinue drug treatment.

Analysis of the medication use process highlights several things. First, the decision by you and other providers to recommend or prescribe drug treatment is a small part of the process. Secondly, patients and professionals may be carrying out parallel decision making with only sporadic communication about these processes. Furthermore, the communication that does occur may be incomplete and ineffective. Yet, both you and your patients may continue making decisions and evaluating outcomes regardless of the quality of understanding of each other's goals, actions, and decisions. One of the aims of the communication process should be to make the patient's understanding and yours regarding the disease, illness experience, and treatment goals as congruent as possible.

It is obvious that there are numerous points in the process where the quality of the patient–professional relationship and the thoroughness of the information exchange affect the decisions of both patients and health professionals. It is at these points that your communication skills are critical and can have the most effect on the outcomes of treatment. As discussed throughout this textbook, you must seize the opportunities in this process when they become available. These opportunities will occur in structured and unstructured environments, in a variety of practice settings, and using varying amounts of time. The key is to maximize patient outcomes by using patient-centered communication skills.

Summary

In establishing effective relationships with patients, your responsibility to help patients achieve desired outcomes must be kept in mind. The patient is the focus of the medication use process. Your communication skills can facilitate formation of trusting relationships with patients. Such a relationship fosters an open exchange of information and a sense of "partnership" between you and your patients. An effective communication process can optimize the chance that patients will make informed decisions, use medications appropriately, and, ultimately, meet therapeutic goals.

REVIEW QUESTIONS

1. **What is patient-centered care?**
2. **What are the two primary functions that the communication process serves between health professionals and patients?**
3. **What is the benefit of analyzing the medication use process from the point of view of patients?**

REVIEW CASES

REVIEW CASE STUDY 1.1

A family who often comes to your pharmacy is facing a devastating situation. The husband lost his minimum-wage job. They were evicted from their apartment, have no extended family to turn to for help, and have a child with asthma who requires medications and ongoing care. The child got a new prescription for a Flovent HFA (1 puff BID) inhaler and Proventil HFA (1 to 2 puffs prn q4–6h) that the family cannot afford.

1. What sources of assistance are available in your community for the housing needs of such a family?
2. What sources of assistance are available for medical and prescription needs?

REVIEW CASE STUDY 1.2

Your patient, Mr. Rowe, is a 65-year-old man who has osteoarthritis. For many years, his hips have hurt him off and on. On days when he experienced pain, he would take one dose of 400 mg of ibuprofen, and that managed the pain. Gradually over the years, the pain became more frequent, and the ibuprofen did not help as much. Then, his knees also began to ache when he went on walks. He talks to you as his pharmacist about how he can manage his pain without having to go to a physician because he does not want to start taking prescription drugs if he can help it.

Question: What further information would you want to obtain from Mr. Rowe that would assist you in deciding how to be of help?

REFERENCES

AHRQ—Agency for Healthcare Research and Quality. *20 Tips to Help Prevent Medical Errors. Patient Fact Sheet*. AHRQ Publication No. 00-PO38. Rockville, MD: Author, 2002.

Beyth RJ, Quinn L, Landefeld CS. A multicomponent intervention to prevent major bleeding complications in older patients receiving warfarin. A randomized, controlled trial. *Annals of Internal Medicine* 133:687–695, 2000.

Bunting BA, Cranor CW. The Asheville Project: Long-term clinical, humanistic, and economic outcomes of a community-based medication therapy management program for asthma. *Journal of the American Pharmacists Association* 46:133–147, 2006.

Centers for Disease Control and Prevention. *Chronic Disease Prevention and Health Promotion*. 2009. Retrieved April 14, 2010 from http://www.cdc.gov/chronicdisease/resources/publications/AAG/chronic.htm.

Committee on Quality of Health Care in America, Institute of Medicine. *To Err is Human—Building a Safer Health System*. Washington, DC: National Academy Press, 1999.

Council on Credentialing for Pharmacy, Scope of Contemporary Pharmacy Practice. *Roles, Responsibilities, and Functions of Pharmacists and Pharmacy Technicians*. Washington, DC: CCP, 2009.

Cox DJ, Gonder-Frederick L, Julian DM, Clarke W. Long-term follow-up evaluation of blood glucose awareness training. *Diabetes Care* 17:1–5, 1994.

Cox DJ, Gonder-Frederick L, Polonsky W, et al. Blood glucose awareness training (BGAT-2): Long-term benefits. *Diabetes Care* 24:637–642, 2001.

Cranor CW, Bunting BA, Christensen DB. The Asheville Project: Long-term clinical and economic outcomes of a community pharmacy diabetes care program. *Journal of the American Pharmacists Association* 43:173–184, 2003.

Darkins A, Ryan P, Kobb R, et al. Care coordination/home telehealth: The systematic implementation of health informatics, home telehealth, and disease management to support the care of veteran patients with chronic conditions. *Telemedicine Journal and E-Health* 14(10):1118–1126, 2008.

Easton KL, Chapman CB, Brien JA. Frequency and characteristics of hospital admissions associated with drug-related problems in paediatrics. *British Journal of Clinical Pharmacology* 57:611–615, 2004.

Ernst FR, Grizzle AJ. Drug-related morbidity and mortality: Updating the cost-of-illness model. *Journal of the American Pharmacists Association* 41:192–199, 2001.

Fallik D. *Drug patch safety triggers an FDA probe*. Philadelphia Inquirer, March 5, 2006. Retrieved May 5, 2006 from http://www.philly.com/mld/philly/living/health/14018264.htm

Field TS, Gilman BH, Subramanian S, et al. The costs associated with adverse drug events among older adults in the ambulatory setting. *Medical Care* 43(12):1171–1176, 2005.

George J, Kong DC, Thoman R, Stewart K. Factors associated with medication nonadherence in patients with COPD. *Chest* 128:3198–3204, 2005.

Greenfield S, Kaplan SH, Ware FE. Expanding patient involvement in care: Effects on patient outcomes. *Annals of Internal Medicine* 102:520–528, 1985.

Greenfield S, Kaplan SH, Ware FE. Patient participation in medical care: Effects on blood sugar and quality of life in diabetes. *Journal of General Internal Medicine* 3:448–457, 1988.

Gurwitz JH, Field TS, Harrold LR, et al. Incidence and preventability of adverse drug events among older persons in the ambulatory setting. *Journal of the American Medical Association* 289: 1107–1116, 2003.

Heath KV, Singer J, O'Shaughnessy MV, et al. Intentional nonadherence due to adverse symptoms associated with antiretroviral therapy. *The Journal of Acquired Immune Deficiency Syndromes* 31:211–217, 2002.

Hepler CD. Regulating for outcomes as a systems response to the problem of drug-related morbidity. *Journal of the American Pharmacists Association* 41:108–115, 2001.

Hepler CD, Strand LM. Opportunities and responsibilities in pharmaceutical care. *American Journal of Hospital Pharmacy* 47:533–543, 1990.

Hickson GB, Clayton EW, Githens PB, et al. Factors that prompted families to file medical malpractice claims following perinatal injuries. *Journal of the American Medical Association* 267:1359–1363, 1992.

ISMP—Institute for Safe Medication Practices. *Medication Safety Alert*. 3(4), April 2004. Retrieved February 23, 2011 from http://www.ismp.org/Newsletters/ambulatory/Issues/community200404.pdf

ISMP—Institute for Safe Medication Practices. *Medication Safety Alert*. 2010 . Retrieved February 23, 2011 from http://www.ismp.org/Newsletters/consumer/alerts/chewable.asp

Joint Commission on Accreditation of Healthcare Organizations . *Five Steps to Safer Healthcare*. Washington, DC: JCAHO, 2002.

Joint Commission of Pharmacy Practitioners. *Future Vision of Pharmacy Practice*. Washington, DC: JCPP, 2008.

Kaplan SH, Greenfield S, Ware JE. Assessing the effects of physician-patient interactions on the outcomes of chronic disease. *Medical Care* 27:S110–S127, 1989.

Kimberlin C, Assa M, Rubin D, Zaenger P. Questions elderly patients have about on-going therapy: A pilot study to assist in communication with physicians. *Pharmacy World and Science* 23: 237–241, 2001.

Kinnaird D, Cox T, Wilson JP. Unclaimed prescriptions in a clinic with computerized prescriber order entry. *American Journal of Health-System Pharmacy* 60:1468–1470, 2003.

Krähenbühl-Melcher A, Schlienger R, Lampert M, et al. Drug-related problems in hospitals: A review of the recent literature. *Drug Safety* 30(5):379–407, 2007.

Leape LL, Cullen DJ, Clapp MD, et al. Pharmacist participation on physician rounds and adverse drug events in the intensive care unit. *Journal of the American Medical Association* 282:267–270, 1999.

Lowry KP, Dudley TK, Oddone EZ, Bosworth HB. Intentional and unintentional nonadherence to antihypertensive medication. *Annals of Pharmacotherapy* 39:1198–1203, 2005.

Mead N, Bower P. Patient-centredness: A conceptual framework and review of the empirical literature. *Social Science and Medicine* 51:1087–1110, 2000.

NCPIE—National Council on Patient Information and Education and the Agency for Healthcare Research and Quality. *Your Medicine: Play it Safe*. Retrieved May 5, 2006 from http://www.talkaboutrx.org/assocdocs/TASK/19/playitsafe_bro.pdf

Olson LM, Tang SF, Newacheck PW. Children in the United States with discontinuous health insurance coverage. *New England Journal of Medicine* 353:382–391, 2005.

Pai AB, Boyd A, Depczynski J, et al. Reduced drug use and hospitalization rates in patients undergoing hemodialysis who received pharmaceutical care: A 2-year, randomized, controlled study. *Pharmacotherapy* 29(12):1433–1440, 2009.

Piette J, Heisler M, Wagner T. Cost-related medication underuse among chronically ill adults: The treatments people forgo, how often, and who is at risk. *American Journal of Public Health* 94(10):1782–1787, 2004.

Piette J, Heisler M, Horne R, Alexander G. A conceptually based approach to understanding chronically ill patients' responses to medication cost pressures. *Social Science & Medicine* 62:846–857, 2006.

Pound P, Britten N, Morgan M, et al. Resisting medicines: A synthesis of qualitative studies of medicine taking. *Social Science & Medicine* 61(1):133–155, 2005.

Reed M, Hargraves L. *Prescription drug access among working-age Americans*. Washington, DC: Center for Studying Health System Change. 2003. Retrieved July 14, 2006 from http://hschange.org/CONTENT/637.

Rodriguez-Monguio R, Otero MJ, Rovira J. Assessing the economic impact of adverse drug effects. *Pharmacoeconomics* 21(9):623–650, 2003.

Rogers S, Wilson D, Wan S, et al. Medication-related admissions in older people: A cross-sectional, observational study. *Drugs Aging* 26(11):951–961, 2009.

Roter DL. Patient question asking in physician-patient interaction. *Health Psychology* 3:395–409, 1984.

Ryan F, Byrne S, O'Shea S. Randomized controlled trial of supervised patient self-testing of warfarin therapy using an Internet-based expert system. *Journal of Thrombosis and Haemostasis* 7(8):1284–1290, 2009.

Safran DG, Neuman P, Schoen C, et al. Prescription drug coverage and seniors: Findings from a 2003 national survey. *Health Affairs* Suppl Web Exclusives: W5-152–W5-166, 2005.

Schachinger H, Hegar K, Hermanns N, et al. Randomized controlled clinical trial of Blood Glucose Awareness Training (BGAT III) in Switzerland and Germany. *Journal of Behavioral Medicine* 28:587–594, 2005.

Schnipper JL, Kirwin JL, Cotugno MC, et al. Role of pharmacist counseling in preventing adverse drug events after hospitalization. *Archives of Internal Medicine* 166:565–571, 2006.

Soumerai S, Pierre-Jacques M, Zhang F, et al. Cost-related medication nonadherence among elderly and disabled Medicare beneficiaries. *Archives of Internal Medicine* 166:1829–1835, 2006.

Spector RA. Plaintiff's attorneys share perspectives on patient communication. *Journal of Healthcare Risk Management* 29(3):29–33, 2010.

Weingart SN, Gandhi TK, Seger AC, et al. Patient-reported medication symptoms in primary care. *Archives of Internal Medicine* 165:234–240, 2005.

Westerlund T, Marklund B. Assessment of the clinical and economic outcomes of pharmacy interventions in drug-related problems. *Journal of Clinical Pharmacy and Therapeutics* 34(3):319–327, 2009.

Wroe AL. Intentional and unintentional nonadherence: A study of decision making. *Journal of Behavioral Medicine* 25:355–372, 2002.

CHAPTER

2

Principles and Elements of Interpersonal Communication

Overview

Interpersonal communication is a common but complex practice that is essential in dealing with patients and other health care providers. This chapter describes the process of interpersonal communication as it relates to pharmacy practice and helps determine what happens when one person tries to express an idea or exchange information with another individual. The information given here is the foundation for subsequent chapters that more fully describe strategies for improving interpersonal relationships and communication.

Setting the Stage

In our personal and professional lives, we need to interact with many people. Some of these interactions are successful, while others are not. Consider Case Study 2.1.

PERSONAL REFLECTION

In most communication encounters, we typically do not have the opportunity to stop and analyze the situation. However, to improve our communication skills, we need some ability to assess a particular situation quickly. Thus, for Case Study 2.1, take a moment now, and on a sheet of paper briefly describe what Mr. Raymond might be thinking or feeling. What clues do you have? Write down what you might say to him. Set the paper aside and read on. Once you have finished the chapter, come back to your notes and rewrite your response based on any insights that resulted from your reading.

CASE STUDY 2.1

George Raymond, a 59-year-old man with moderate hypertension, enters your pharmacy holding an unlit cigar. You know George because you attend the same church. He is a high school principal, has a wife who works, and has four children. He has been told to quit smoking and go on a diet. He also has a long history of not taking his medications correctly. He comes to pick up a new prescription—an antibiotic for a urinary tract infection. Although he knows you personally, he is somewhat hesitant as he approaches the counseling area. He looks down at the ground and mumbles, "The doctor called in a new prescription for me, and can I also have a refill of my heart medication?"

Components of the Interpersonal Communication Model

Communication encompasses a broad spectrum of media, for example, mass communication (TV, radio), small-group communication (committee meetings, discussion groups), and large-group communication (lectures, speeches). This book will not address these types of communication, but will focus on one-to-one interpersonal communication that occurs in pharmacy practice, such as that observed in the situation with George Raymond. In this section, the interpersonal communication process, or the interaction between two individuals, will be described in detail. This specific form of communication (interpersonal communication) is best described as a process in which messages are generated and transmitted by one person and subsequently received and translated by another. A practical model of this process is shown in Figure 2-1. This model builds on the original work of Shannon and Weaver (1949). The model includes five important elements: sender, message, receiver, feedback, and barriers.

THE SENDER

In the interpersonal communication process, the sender transmits a message to another person. In the example described above, the initial sender of a message was Mr. Raymond: "The doctor called in a new prescription for me, and can I also have a refill of my heart medication?"

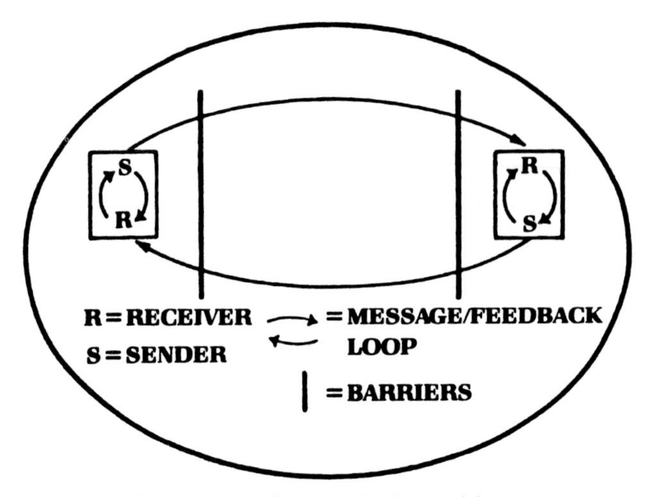

FIGURE 2-1. The interpersonal communication model.

THE MESSAGE

In interpersonal communication, the message is the element that is transmitted from one person to another. Messages can be thoughts, ideas, emotions, information, or other factors and can be transmitted both verbally (by talking) and nonverbally (by using facial expressions, hand gestures, and so on). For example, Mr. Raymond's verbal message was that he wanted his new prescription and that he would like to have his prescription for heart medication refilled. At the same time, he also communicated nonverbal messages. Did you recognize any of these nonverbal messages? By looking down at the ground and mumbling rather than speaking clearly, he might have been expressing embarrassment, shyness, or hesitancy to talk with you. He might have felt embarrassed, perhaps because he had not been taking his heart pills regularly. As discussed in greater detail in Chapter 3, the nonverbal component of communication is important. Research has found that in some situations 55% or more of the meaning of a message is transmitted through its nonverbal component.

In most situations, senders formulate (encode) messages before transmitting them. However, in some cases, messages are transmitted spontaneously without the sender thinking about them, such as a glaring stare or a burst of laughter. In the earlier situation, Mr. Raymond may not have been aware that he was transmitting nonverbal messages to you.

THE RECEIVER

The receiver (you in the above example) receives the message from the sender (Mr. Raymond). As the receiver, you "decode" the message and assign a particular meaning to it, which may or may not be Mr. Raymond's intended meaning. In receiving and translating the message, you probably considered both the verbal and nonverbal components of the messages sent by Mr. Raymond.

FEEDBACK

Feedback is the process whereby receivers communicate back to senders their understanding of the sender's message. In most situations, receivers do not passively absorb messages; they respond to them with their own verbal and nonverbal messages. By using verbal and nonverbal communication, the receiver feeds back information to the sender about how the message was translated. In the feedback loop, the initial receiver becomes the sender of feedback, and the initial sender becomes the receiver of feedback, as noted in the model. In the interpersonal communication process, individuals are thus constantly moving back and forth between the roles of sender and receiver. In the earlier example, you were first a receiver of information from Mr. Raymond; when you responded to him with a statement, such as "So you want your medication refilled?" you became a sender of feedback to Mr. Raymond.

Feedback can be simple, such as merely nodding your head, or more complex, such as repeating a set of complicated instructions to make sure that you interpreted them correctly. In your Personal Reflection, how did you respond to Mr. Raymond? You could have said, "I'm sorry, George, I'm not sure what you are asking. Which medication do you need?" or "How are you feeling, George? You seem a bit down." Thus, in this example, feedback would be your verbal and nonverbal response to Mr. Raymond. Feedback allows communication to be a two-way interaction rather than a one-way monologue.

During the communication process, most of us tend to focus on the message and frequently miss the opportunity for feedback. As receivers of messages, we fail to provide appropriate feedback to the sender about our understanding of the message. On the other hand, as senders of messages, we fail to ask for feedback from the receiver, or in some cases ignore feedback provided by others. Consequently, we are led to think that a particular communication interaction was more effective than it really was (i.e., "I really felt she understood what I told her."). As discussed in Chapter 5, being sensitive to others can strengthen our ability to receive and provide useful feedback.

BARRIERS

Interpersonal communication is usually affected by a number of interferences or barriers. These barriers affect the accuracy of the communication exchange. For example, if a loud vacuum cleaner was running in your pharmacy when you are trying to talk to Mr. Raymond, it may be difficult to understand what he was trying to communicate. Other barriers to your interaction with Mr. Raymond might include a safety glass partition between you and Mr. Raymond, telephones ringing in the background, or Mr. Raymond's inability to hear you due to his defective hearing aid. Barriers can be so detrimental to interpersonal communication that we will devote an entire chapter (see Chapter 4) to strategies for identifying and then minimizing possible communication barriers (see Figure 2-2).

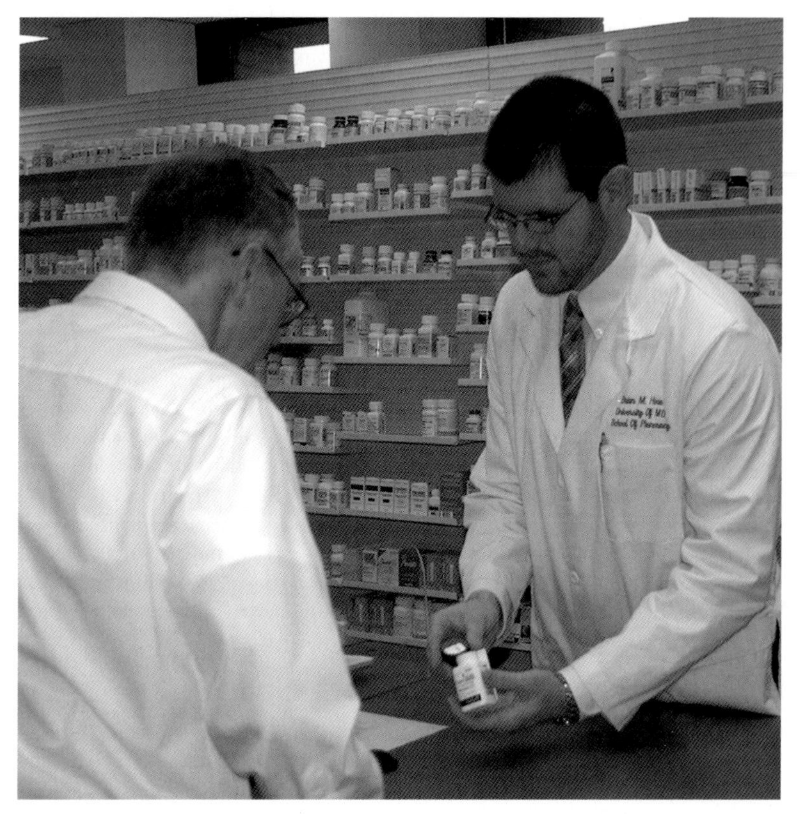

FIGURE 2-2. In this counseling situation, what is the pharmacist doing correctly? What needs to be improved?

Personal Responsibilities in the Communication Model

The model presented in Figure 2-1 is useful because it is easy to understand, but it does oversimplify the communication process. In any interpersonal communication situation, individuals at any point in time are simultaneously sending and receiving messages. For example, in the scenario described above, the initial spoken message was sent by Mr. Raymond: "The doctor called in a new prescription for me, and can I also have a refill of my heart medication?" However, at the time that he was speaking to you, he was probably observing your nonverbal behaviors and so was receiving messages from you as he was sending the verbal message. He was probably noticing whether you were paying attention, whether you were smiling, whether you acknowledged receipt of his spoken messages by nodding your head, and so on. Individuals cannot be in the presence of another person without both sending and receiving messages, regardless of who is speaking. Even if nothing is spoken, the silence is interpreted. For example, if a new patient receives a prescription from a pharmacy assistant within sight of the pharmacist but the pharmacist does not speak, the patient may interpret the pharmacist's silence to mean that he does not want to talk to the patient. All communication is transactional, and the interaction includes both verbal and nonverbal messages.

As a sender, you are responsible for ensuring that the message is transmitted in the clearest form, in terminology understood by the other person, and in an environment conducive to clear transmission. To check whether the message was received as intended, you need to ask for feedback from the receiver and clarify any misunderstandings. Thus, your obligation as the sender of a message is not complete until you have determined that the other person has understood the message correctly.

As a receiver, you have the responsibility of listening to what is transmitted by the sender. To ensure accurate communication, you should provide feedback to the sender by describing what you understood the message to be. Many times, we feel that feedback is not necessary because we assume that we understand each other completely. However, practice has found that without appropriate feedback, misunderstandings occur. Of concern is that, as pharmacists dealing with patients, physicians, and other health care providers, we cannot afford these misunderstandings. These misunderstandings might result in harm to the patient. To become more effective, efficient, and accurate in our communication, we must strive to include explicit feedback in our interactions with others.

In Search of the Meaning of the Message

The interpersonal communication model shows how messages originate from a sender and are received by a receiver. The sender delivers the message, and the receiver assigns a meaning to that message. The critical component in this process is that the receiver's assigned meaning must be the same as the meaning intended by the sender. In other words, we may or may not interpret the meaning of the various verbal and nonverbal messages in the same way as the sender intended. For example, in the encounter with Mr. Raymond, you may have inferred that since he was looking down at the ground that he was embarrassed or hesitant to talk with you. However, he may have been looking down at a coffee stain on the new tie that his wife gave him. He may have been upset at himself for being so clumsy and not really concerned about what messages he was sending you. Thus, the message that you received might not have been the one Mr. Raymond intended to send.

WORDS AND THEIR CONTEXT

In general, individuals assign meaning to verbal and nonverbal messages based on their past experiences and previous definitions of these verbal and nonverbal elements. If two persons do not share the same definitions or past experiences, misunderstanding may occur. The most common example of this is evident in different languages and dialects of the world. Different words mean different things to different people based on the definitions learned. For example, "football" to an American means a sport using an oval ball, but "football" to a European means a sport using a round ball (soccer). An example of this misunderstanding occurs in health care when we speak in medical terminology that may have different (or possibly no) meaning to our patients. The following example illustrates this potential misunderstanding.

In the beginning exercise, let us assume that you wish to inform Mr. Raymond that his urinary tract antibiotic will be more effective if taken with sufficient fluid to guarantee adequate urinary output. You relate that intent in the following manner, "This medication should be taken with plenty of fluids." The message is received and decoded into words and symbols in the mind of Mr. Raymond. These words or symbols may or may not have any particular meaning to him. Perhaps he does not know what "fluids" refers to; perhaps he is uncertain whether you consider milk to be a fluid. Perhaps he associates the word "plenty" with a small glass of orange juice at breakfast rather than the 8-ounce glass of water that you had in mind. Thus, the meaning of your important message may or may not have been received accurately by Mr. Raymond. It is the assignment of meaning to your words by Mr. Raymond that is important.

Another important factor is that people assign meanings based on the context that they perceive the sender is using. Often patients assign different meanings to our messages than the ones we intended. The actual situation described in Case Study 2.2 illustrates this point.

In this example, the mother understood the words on the label, but she put them into a different context and thus derived a different meaning from the one intended. Apparently, the original pharmacist did not have the opportunity to talk with the mother when she picked up the antibiotic prescription to ask her how she was going to give the medication to her son. In other words, the pharmacist did not ask for feedback from the mother on how she interpreted the message on the label.

CASE STUDY 2.2

A 9-month-old baby is admitted to the hospital with a severe infection. You, the pharmacist, speak with the mother upon admission and learn that about 1 week ago, her son had developed a minor bacterial infection and received an antibiotic. The mother stopped giving her baby the antibiotic after 4 days of therapy (rather than the necessary 10 days) because it appeared that the infection was cured. When you asked her why she stopped the antibiotic, the mother stated that she was just following the directions on the prescription label: "Take one-half teaspoonful three times a day for infection until all gone." The mother stated that she gave the medication until the infection was "all gone." Unfortunately, the intended message was that the antibiotic should have been given until the liquid was all gone. The mother assigned a meaning to the message on the prescription label that was not accurate; thus, she stopped giving the antibiotic, a superinfection developed, and the baby was hospitalized.

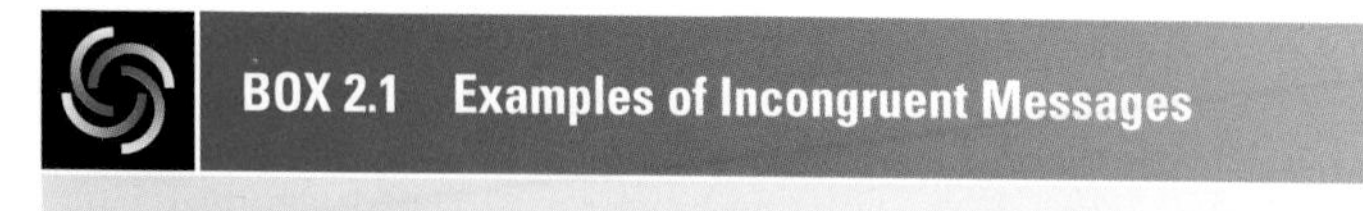

BOX 2.1 Examples of Incongruent Messages

- A red-faced agitated patron comes into the pharmacy, raises a fist, and loudly proclaims, "I'm not angry, I'm just here to ask about a prescription error."
- A disappointed pharmacist has tried, so far without success, to convince a physician to change an obviously inappropriate medication order. When asked how he is feeling, he meekly replies, "Oh, I'm just fine."
- A patient hands a pharmacist a prescription for a tranquilizer, then bursts into tears. The pharmacist asks if anything is the matter, and the patient responds, "No, I'm okay, it's nothing at all."

The social context also influences how messages are received and interpreted. The type of relationship that patients have with you determines the level of acceptance that patients have regarding the information provided. Research has shown that if patients perceive pharmacists to be credible, unbiased providers of useful information, they will listen and retain more information about their medications. If they perceive pharmacists to be trustworthy and honest, they will be more willing to approach pharmacists for assistance.

CONGRUENCE BETWEEN VERBAL AND NONVERBAL MESSAGES

The meaning of the message may be somewhat unclear if the receiver senses incongruence between the verbal and nonverbal messages. That is, the meaning of a verbal message is not consistent with the meaning of a nonverbal message. The situations depicted in Box 2.1 reveal potentially incongruent messages.

In each of these examples, the verbal message obviously did not match the nonverbal message, and the receiver may be confused about the true message intended by the sender. To avoid this incongruence, as a sender, you must be aware of the nonverbal messages as well as the verbal messages. As a receiver, you must point out to the sender that you are receiving two different messages.

In summary, people base their interpretation of verbal and nonverbal messages on a variety of factors. These factors include their definitions and perceptions of the words, symbols, and nonverbal elements used by the sender. In reality, the final message is not what is said, but what the receiver perceives was said. The following section discusses how to prevent potential misunderstandings.

PREVENTING MISUNDERSTANDING

In the previous situation involving the baby's antibiotic prescription, the label read, "Take one-half teaspoonful three times a day for infection until all gone." Unfortunately, the mother interpreted the message incorrectly. In this situation, the meaning could be clarified relatively easily by rearranging the position of the last two prepositional phrases (…three times a day until all medication is finished for infection) or rearranging the wording (…until the medication is all gone). However, minimizing misunderstandings is many times more difficult in other situations. We often assume that the receiver will interpret our message accurately. To improve the communication process, we must remember that people assign meanings to messages based on their background, values, and experiences. If other persons have different backgrounds, values, and experiences, they may assign a different meaning to our intended message. Many of our problems in communication occur because we forget that individual experiences are never identical. In actual practice, we have enough common experiences with people we deal with on a daily basis that we can understand each other fairly well.

Often we can anticipate patients' feelings and their understanding about the use of medications. Communication breaks down when we have limited common experiences or do not share the same meaning of certain words and symbols. Thus, a person placed on a medication for the first time has a different perception than a person who has taken the medication for several years, or a person of a different gender, age, or race may have experiences different from ours.

A key to preventing misunderstanding is anticipating how other people may translate your message. It may be helpful to determine their experience with medications in general and with a particular medication specifically. If they have had positive experiences previously, their perception of medications may be different than if they have had negative experiences. If they have negative feelings about medications, they may be reluctant to discuss the medication or even to take it. We need to ask certain questions to determine these perceptions. What do you already know about this medication? How do you feel about taking this medication? Some of the skills discussed in Chapter 5 on empathic listening may be helpful in anticipating how others may assign meaning to your message. In many communication interactions, the more you know about other people and the more you are able to understand them, the easier it will be to anticipate how they may interpret the meaning of the message.

USING FEEDBACK TO CHECK THE MEANING OF THE MESSAGE

Predicting how a person will translate a particular message is difficult. Using a technique described earlier (providing feedback to check the meaning of the message) may alleviate some communication misunderstandings. As senders of messages, we should ask others to share their interpretation of the message. In the example of the antibiotic, the original pharmacist should have asked the mother in a nonthreatening manner, "When you get home, how long are you going to give the medication to your son?" Thus, her initial perception could have been corrected, and the problem could have been avoided. We typically do not ask for feedback from patrons to check their perceptions of the meaning of our messages. Verifying the fact that the receiver interpreted the intended meaning of our verbal and nonverbal messages accurately takes additional time and is sometimes awkward. Most people rely on their own intuition as to whether their

CASE STUDY 2.3

A patient being seen in an anticoagulation clinic mentions to you, the pharmacist, that he had developed several bruises on his hands and legs. You immediately check the patient's computer records and find a recent INR value of 6 which is well above his targeted 2 to 3 range. You ask if the patient has changed his diet, lifestyle, or medication regimen. The patient says no, but that he was given another medication during his last clinic visit. You then go back to the profile and notice that the patient has been receiving 4 mg daily Coumadin for some time, but his dose was reduced to 3 mg during the last visit to adjust his INR. You suspect what the issue might be and ask the patient, "Did you stop taking the 4-mg tablet?" The patient replies, "No, nobody told me to, so I have been following instructions and taking both tablets!" Thus, he was taking 7 mg per day rather than the intended 3 mg!

intended message was received correctly. Case Study 2.3 illustrates the harmful effects of not asking for feedback from patients on how they intend to take the medication.

Unfortunately, relying on our intuition is not as effective as obtaining explicit feedback to measure understanding. Examples of how to ask for feedback are shown in Box 2.2. The preceding paragraphs describe ways to minimize misunderstanding from the sender's perspective. However, the receiver can also alleviate some misunderstanding by offering feedback to the sender. After receiving the message, you should indicate in some way what you understand the message to be. It is particularly important for you to provide feedback by summarizing the information you have received from patients in the course of interviews conducted or assessments made related to their drug therapy. Since you are primarily the "receiver" when obtaining information from patients on their symptoms or current therapy, you should provide feedback to verify your understanding. When you are primarily the "sender," as when you give information on a new

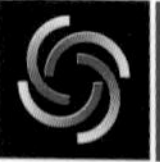

BOX 2.2 Statements or Questions That Elicit Feedback

- "I want to be sure I have explained things clearly. Please summarize the most important things to remember about this medicine."
- "How do you intend to take the medication?"
- "Please show me how you are going to use this nasal inhaler."
- "Describe in your own words how you are going to take this medication."

prescription, then the patient should be asked to summarize key information presented as a way of providing feedback that your message was understood accurately. In later chapters, specific skills are offered as means of improving your ability to give feedback and receive feedback from others.

Importance of Perception in Communication

Perception is important in the process of interpersonal communication because we tend to interpret messages based on our perception of (1) what we believe the message says and (2) the individual sending the message. Thus, perceptual barriers need to be identified and minimized, or we will misinterpret what we hear. We need to recognize how fragile the communication process is during professional communication and to value the use of feedback to enhance our ability to verify the true meaning of messages.

PERCEPTION OF MEANINGS WITHIN A MESSAGE

People assign meanings to verbal and nonverbal messages based on their perception of the intended meaning (Fabun, 1986). In other words, the receiver's perception of the words, symbols, and nonverbal elements used by the sender influences how the receiver interprets the meaning. It is not what is said, but what the receiver perceives to have been said. The actual situation in Case Study 2.4 illustrates this point.

The patient perceived the phrase "apply one daily" to be absolute, so he applied one each day (but did not perceive the implied message that he should remove one). He followed his perception of the instructions. Unfortunately, no one asked him how he was going to use the patches (in other words, did not ask for feedback on his perception of the instructions). If the original pharmacist had verified the patient's understanding, the patient would have been spared the resulting embarrassment and resulting side effects. Misperceptions like this occur frequently in pharmacy practice, and most pharmacists have a story to tell about how patients misuse medications based on their misperceptions. The outcomes of these situations can be quite serious as noted in Case Studies 2.4 and 2.5.

CASE STUDY 2.4

A patient returns to your pharmacy complaining of side effects apparently caused by his new medication. The patient's records indicated he was given 30 nitroglycerin patches about 1 month ago. Both the original pharmacist and the physician told him to "apply one daily," which is a typical dose for this type of patient. You ask him, "What seems to be the problem?" He states, "I don't feel too good and I am running out of room" and then opens his shirt to reveal 27 nitroglycerin patches firmly adhered to his chest!

CASE STUDY 2.5

A young woman suffering from vaginal candidiasis was given seven vaginal tablets and was told by the pharmacist to "use one tablet daily for 1 week." She returned to the pharmacy after 3 days in severe discomfort with a complaint that "Those tablets taste terrible!"

In this example, the patient assigned the wrong meaning to the word "use" and used the medication the way she typically uses medications—by taking them orally. She acted based on her perceptions that were influenced by her past experiences and background; perceptions that were not corrected by the original pharmacist. The challenge facing you in practice is that it is difficult to recognize when your patients have different perceptions than you.

One skill that minimizes perceptual differences is to use terms and concepts that are familiar to the patient. It is very easy for patients to misunderstand when you use abstract terms, such as "Drink a lot of fluid." What does "a lot" mean to a patient? A glass? A cup? Broad, nonspecific directions do not help patients understand what you want to communicate. Another example might be, instead of asking patients if they "hurt a lot," you should ask them, "Describe your pain on a scale of 0 to 10 with 0 being no pain and 10 being the worst pain imaginable." You should also avoid using professional jargon. For example, most people are not impressed by the fact that they have "intermittent claudication," when all they want is help with their inability to walk any distance without experiencing leg pain. You must also recognize gender differences and cultural differences (discussed further in Chapter 10) that may lead to misperceptions.

PERCEPTIONS OF INDIVIDUALS

Our perception of the message is also influenced by our perception of the individual sending the message (Keltner, 1970). How we perceive the sender affects the interpretation of the message. We respond using our perception of that individual as our reference point because we tend to be influenced by a person's cultural background, status, gender, or age. These perceptions are further influenced by any bias we have or stereotypes we hold of certain groups of individuals. The following statements illustrate this point:

"People who are mentally ill do not comply with their medication regimens."
"Nurses always complain about pharmacists."
"Elderly people can't hear well and always talk too much."
"People who talk slow are lazy."
"Women with red hair have a temper."

We do not see the person as a unique individual but as a representative of a particular group (e.g., elderly, mentally ill, etc.). We erect "perceptual barriers" to the communication process not based on fact but on our inferences based on stereotypes. Unfortunately, these barriers inhibit true communication between individuals.

We need to evaluate when our perception of the sender is incorrect or when our assumptions might be interfering with our ability to communicate with others. We may need to "check" our assumption before proceeding. Does the elderly person really have a hearing deficiency? Does the person who talks slowly have a learning disability? Increased awareness of stereotyping and additional effort in checking our assumptions can enhance our interpersonal communication.

Unfortunately, the people you deal with on a daily basis may have perceptions of you as a pharmacist that interfere with your ability to communicate with them. Their perceptions may not be based on reality but on their stereotypes of pharmacists. Patient perceptions are influenced by their past experiences with pharmacists, by what others have said about pharmacists, or by what they have read in magazines and newspapers. For example, patients may perceive you as an uncaring, busy person who is concerned only with filling prescriptions and taking their money. These stereotypes influence what they may say to you and how they may listen to you. If they perceive you as a professional, they will listen to what you tell them about their medications. By the same token, if nurses, physicians, and other health care providers do not perceive you as a professional, they will not value the information you provide. Part of improving communication with others is to determine what their perceptions of pharmacists are and then try to alter those perceptions if they are unfounded. Additional examples of perceptual barriers are provided in Chapter 10 during the discussion of cultural competence.

SHARING THE SAME PERCEPTIONS

One key to preventing misunderstanding is to try to understand and share the perceptions of other individuals (Applebaum et al., 1985). Many times, using "lay language," which is familiar to patients, rather than medical terminology, which is familiar only to health care professionals, can enhance understanding. Determining the patient's past experience with medications or with the particular drugs prescribed may also be helpful. Patients who have had positive experiences previously may be more willing to take the medication. However, if their past experiences have been bad, they may be reluctant to even begin taking the medication.

Frequently, it is difficult to understand patient backgrounds and to predict perceptions of the messages you may provide (see Box 2.3). Some of the skills discussed in Chapter 5 on empathic listening may be helpful. In many communication interactions, the more you know about the other person and the more they can know about you, the easier it is to share the same perception.

USING FEEDBACK TO VERIFY PERCEPTIONS

The best technique to alleviate harmful misperceptions is using feedback to verify the perceived meaning of a message. As a sender of messages, you should ask others to share their interpretations of the message. In the nitroglycerin example,

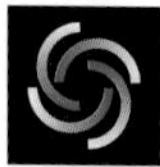

BOX 2.3 Advice Pharmacists Should Follow When Communicating with People of Different Backgrounds

- Learn as much as you can about the patient's background, including beliefs about taking medications.
- View diversity as an opportunity. With a little patience and the right attitude, you will be amazed at the opportunities that crop up to help one another.
- Do not condescend. Patronizing behavior is not appreciated and is recognized as such in any culture.
- Talk about your differences. Misunderstandings will often take root when people from differing backgrounds do not talk to one another. Be willing to talk openly and with a constructive attitude.

the pharmacist should have asked the patient in a nonthreatening manner how he was going to use the patches. We typically do not ask for feedback from patients to check their perceptions of the words used when we give directions. We simply assume that patients understand us. Just think how many medication misadventures could be prevented if pharmacists would have asked patients to give them feedback using this phrase, "Before you leave, could you please tell me how you are going to use this medicine?"

The receiver can also alleviate some misunderstanding by offering feedback to the sender. After receiving the message, receivers should summarize the key elements of the message. In later chapters, specific skills are offered to improve your ability to give feedback and to receive feedback from others.

Summary

The interpersonal communication model reveals that you must recognize that interpersonal communication is more than merely speaking to others, offering a printed prescription label, or handing the patient a medication information leaflet. You must make sure that the messages you transmit to others are received accurately. There is no guarantee that the meaning of your message will be translated as intended. You need to make sure you enhance your listening skills so that you can become a better receiver of messages as well.

In the remaining chapters, we provide practical skills necessary for improving your communication. Each chapter builds on the preceding one. Communication is a complex process that may be difficult for some. However, it is a process that can be easily managed and controlled like any other learned skill. By emphasizing practical applications, we hope to lower any barriers that you may have to improving the valuable skills involved in communicating effectively. Before going further, go back and reread your comments about Mr. Raymond's situation, and see if there is anything that you would do differently.

REVIEW QUESTIONS

1. **Describe the five components in the communications model.**
2. **Where do the meanings of messages come from?**
3. **What happens when verbal and nonverbal messages are not congruent?**
4. **What is meant by "Our perception of a message is affected by our perception of the individual"?**
5. **How can misperceptions be minimized?**

REVIEW CASES

REVIEW CASE STUDY 2.1

A patient, Ms. Reynolds, enters a pharmacy having just come from her physician's office.

Ms. Reynolds: My doctor just gave me a prescription for methotrexate and did not tell me anything about it! What's it used for?

Pharmacist: I am kind of busy right now to go into detail, but it is used to treat various conditions including cancer.

Ms. Reynolds: Cancer! My doctor didn't say anything about cancer.

1. How could have the pharmacist handled this situation differently to check for misperceptions?
2. What would you have said to the patient?
3. Would you call anyone else about this? If so, who?

REVIEW CASE STUDY 2.2

You are a pharmacist in a pharmacy located in a medical building. Cynthia Jackson, a 22-year-old college student, enters your pharmacy. Cynthia has no prescription insurance and is on a limited budget. She has been dealing with chronic sinusitis and finally realized that she needed to see an ear, nose, and throat specialist. Cynthia visited Dr. Sampson, who practices in your building.

REVIEW CASE STUDY 2.2, Cont.

You know Dr. Sampson to be a good physician, but one who lacks interpersonal skills at times. He prescribed an expensive antibiotic that would cost Cynthia $75. After you tell her the price, Cynthia states: "Dr. Sampson didn't help me very much. He spends 5 minutes with me and then prescribes this expensive antibiotic and nothing else! And how can a simple antibiotic cost so much?"

1. What feelings do you sense coming from Cynthia?
2. How does Cynthia's perception of Dr. Sampson influence her behavior?
3. How would you respond to Cynthia?
4. What kind of recommendations would you give her?

REFERENCES

Applebaum RL, Jenson DO, Caroll R. *Speech Communication*. New York, NY: Macmillan, 1985.

Fabun D. *Communications: The Transfer of Meaning*. Toronto: Glencoe Press, 1986.

Keltner SW. *Interpersonal Speech Communication: Elements and Structures*. Belmont, CA: Wadsworth, 1970.

Shannon CE, Weaver W. *The Mathematical Theory of Communication*. Urbana, IL: University of Illinois Press, 1949.

RECOMMENDED READINGS

Beebe SA, Beebe SJ, Redmond MV. *Interpersonal Communication: Relating to Others* (2nd ed.). Boston, MA: Allyn & Bacon, 1999.

Casswell HD. The structure and function of communication in society. In L. Bryson (ed.). *The Communication of Ideas*. New York, NY: Institute for Religion and Social Studies, 1948.

Hargie OD, Morrow NC, Woodman C. Pharmacists' evaluation of key communication skills in practice. *Patient Education and Counseling* 39:61–70, 2000.

Shah BK, Chewning BA. Conceptualizing and measuring pharmacist-patient communication: A review. *Journal of the American Pharmacists Association* 45(2):267, 2005.

Svarstad BL, Bultman DC, Mount JK. Patient counseling provided in community pharmacies: Effects of state regulation, pharmacist age, and busyness. *Journal of the American Pharmacists Association* 44(1):22–29, 2004.

Wood JT. *Interpersonal Communication: Everyday Encounters* (2nd ed.). New York, NY: Wadsworth, 1999.

Worley-Louis MM, Schommer JC, Finnegan JR. Construct identification and measure development for investigating pharmacy-patient relationships. *Patient Education and Counseling* 51:299–238, 2003.

CHAPTER

3

Nonverbal Communication

Overview

Words are not the only way by which pharmacists communicate. Interpersonal communication involves both verbal and nonverbal expression. Words normally express ideas, whereas nonverbal expressions convey attitudes and emotions. A large measure of how you relate to others and how they relate to you is not based on what is said, but on what is not said. You may not speak or even have the desire to communicate, and yet be engaged in a communication process. You are constantly providing "messages" to those around you by your dress, facial expression, body movements, and other aspects of your appearance and behavior. Nonverbal expressions include kinesics, proxemics, and elements of the physical environment in which communication takes place. This chapter describes the various components of nonverbal communication and discusses how it plays an important role in effective patient-centered communication.

Nonverbal Versus Verbal Communication

Nonverbal communication involves a complete mix of behaviors, psychological responses, and environmental interactions through which we consciously or unconsciously relate to another person. It differs from verbal communication in that the medium of exchange is neither vocalized language nor the written word. The importance of nonverbal communication is underlined by the findings of behavioral scientists, who have reported that approximately 55% to 95% of all communication can be attributed to nonverbal sources (Mehrabian, 1971; Poytos, 1983). Awareness and skilled use of your nonverbal abilities can make the difference between fulfilling, successful interpersonal relationships and frustrated, nonproductive interactions.

Nonverbal communications are unique for three reasons. First, they mirror innermost thoughts and feelings. This mirror effect is constantly at work, whether or not you are conscious of it. Second, nonverbal communication is difficult, if not impossible, to "fake" during an interpersonal interaction. Third, your nonverbal communication must be consistent with your verbal communication or people will be suspicious of the intended meaning of your message. This lack of congruence between your verbal and nonverbal messages may result in less than successful interpersonal communication (Borman et al., 1969).

In nonverbal communication, we perceive and interpret a given nonverbal message or "cue" in a personal manner. Various interpretations emerge from the different social, psychological, cultural, and other background variables of the senders and receivers of nonverbal messages. For example, a simple nod of the head or a specific hand gesture may mean something to one person but something completely different to another. Therefore, nonverbal "cues" can and often do have multiple interpretations. However, within a given society, groups of nonverbal cues or "cue clusters" generally result in interpretations that are universally agreed upon.

Cue clusters are combinations of nonverbal acts that communicate certain global messages. For example, a patient who gives you a friendly handshake, a pleasant-sounding "thank you," and a warm smile at the end of your interaction is probably more pleased with the interaction than a patient who abruptly turns around and quickly walks away mumbling something under his breath. Without a doubt, cue clusters contribute significantly to what is being communicated nonverbally. On the other hand, the specific "reasons" behind a person's nonverbal behaviors (e.g., "why" a patient turned abruptly and walked away) usually cannot be determined from the nonverbal communication alone. You may sense that a patient seems upset. However, you do not know whether the cause is distress over something you said, discouragement at being ill, dismay over the cost of the medication, a desire to hurry to get back to work, or a myriad of other things that may be on the patient's mind that would explain his or her behavior. When analyzing nonverbal communication, avoid focusing on just one cue. Look at all the nonverbal cues that you are receiving and use verbal communication to fully understand the meaning of the nonverbal behavior.

Elements of Nonverbal Communication

Important nonverbal elements discussed here include kinesics (body movement), proxemics (distance between persons trying to communicate), the physical

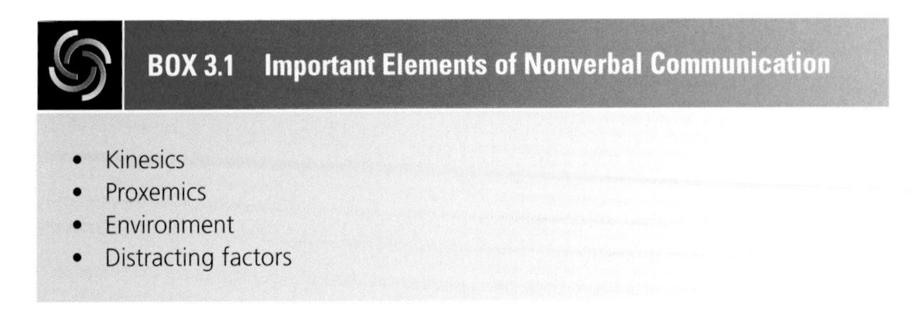

BOX 3.1 Important Elements of Nonverbal Communication

- Kinesics
- Proxemics
- Environment
- Distracting factors

environment, and potential distracting elements of nonverbal communication (see Box 3.1).

KINESICS

The manner in which you use your arms, legs, hands, head, face, and torso may have a dramatic impact on the messages that you send. In general, individuals from various societies use different body movements to communicate certain messages. In this country, for example, it is common for two men to shake hands when meeting each other. A handshake is a way by which we nonverbally indicate friendship or acceptance of the other person. The handshake stems from much earlier times when a man who extended his hand to another was communicating the fact that he held no weapon to do harm. However, in some cultures, it is more appropriate to bow to each other rather than shake each other's hand.

As a health care professional, you need to generate a feeling of empathy and commitment to the helping of others. It is apparent, therefore, that your body movement or kinesics should complement this role. An open stance can nonverbally communicate sincerity, respect, and empathy for another person. The classic example of an open posture is standing (or sitting) with a full frontal appearance to the other person. As an open communicator, you should also have your legs and arms comfortably apart (not crossed) and a facial expression that expresses interest and a desire to listen as well as speak.

A closed posture occurs when you have your arms folded in front of your chest, legs crossed at the knees, head facing downward, and eyes looking away from the patient. If you hold this posture during an interaction, the other person may respond in a similar noncommunicative manner or may break off the interaction altogether. Communication from a closed posture may shorten or halt further productive interactions. Sometimes it is appropriate to use a closed posture, for example, when you want to limit the interaction with an overly talkative person.

The key is to be aware of your tendency to close off communication through your body movements. For example, if during a consultation you suddenly have the impression that the patient is no longer interested in speaking with you, examine your body position to see whether it appears to be defensive. To improve communication kinesics, consider the suggestions in Box 3.2.

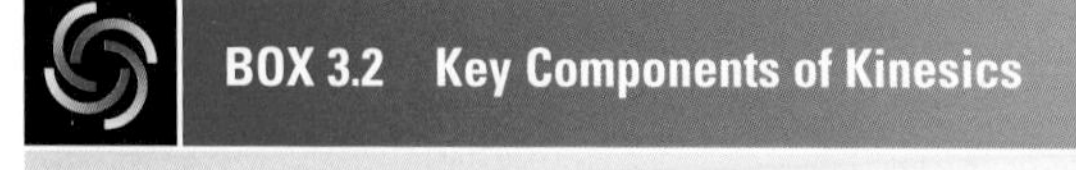

BOX 3.2 Key Components of Kinesics

- Varied eye contact (consistent, but not a stare)
- Relaxed posture
- Appropriate comfortable gestures
- Frontal appearance (shoulders square to other person)
- Slight lean toward the other person
- Erect body position (head up, shoulders back)

PROXEMICS

The distance between two interacting persons plays an important role in nonverbal communication. Proxemics, the structure and use of space, is a powerful nonverbal tool. Behavioral scientists have found that the quality of interactions can vary depending upon the distances between the communicators (Keltner, 1970). In many cultures, people reserve the most protected space (within 18 inches from their bodies) for others with whom they have close, intimate relationships. When someone else ventures into this space during a conversation, people may experience anxiety and perhaps anger at the trespass of their intimate zone. A crowded elevator is the best illustration of the need to maintain intimate space. People in a crowded elevator will do almost anything (to the point of standing like statues) to avoid touching one another. If by chance two people in this situation do have bodily contact, they usually apologize, even though neither person had an opportunity to avoid the trespass of space.

Most people in the United States tend to be more comfortable when a distance of 18 inches to 48 inches is maintained between other individuals. At this distance, casual personal conversations normally take place. Interpersonal distances of more than 4 to 6 feet are generally reserved for public rather than private communication. Further distances would not be appropriate for patient counseling, especially if other individuals are within earshot of the conversation. Thus, you must consider the distance factor whenever you consult with patients. You want to stand close enough to ensure privacy, yet at the same time provide enough room so that the patient feels comfortable. You do not want to invade a patient's intimate zone nor conduct the counseling session in the public zone. Patients usually indicate nonverbally whether they feel comfortable with the distance by either stepping backward or leaning forward.

The type of instructions that you need to give to the patient will also affect the distance. For sensitive issues, such as explaining the use of a rectal or vaginal medication, you may need to enter the patient's private zone, especially if others are around. Ideally, the pharmacy setting should provide various levels of privacy so that both the sender and the receiver of messages feel comfortable.

ENVIRONMENTAL NONVERBAL FACTORS

A number of environmental factors play important roles in communicating nonverbal messages to patients. For example, the colors used in the pharmacy's decor, the lighting, and the uses of space are important nonverbal communication factors. Within the community practice setting, the use of the prescription counter is an important environmental factor. The counter and related shelving serve to keep the prescription dispensing process from the public's view. However, they can also serve as communication barriers if they inhibit your interaction with your patients. When appropriate, step to the side of the prescription counter or from behind the counter to communicate a genuine interest in talking with patients about their medications. In addition, the presence of a private consulting area may indicate to your patients that you are interested in counseling them in a private manner.

The general appearance within the pharmacy setting conveys nonverbal messages to patients. Dirt, clutter, and general untidiness carry negative nonverbal messages. These messages influence patient perceptions about your professional role and your level of interest in serving your patients. For example, counseling around I.V. boxes in a room that doubles as a storage room in an outpatient clinic will likely be perceived by a patient to be a very unprofessional encounter. In addition, the physical characteristics of pharmacy employees also send nonverbal messages to patients. Professional staff should dress appropriately. You want to convey a friendly appearance, but you also want to convey professional competence. Your appearance and the appearance of your fellow employees can enhance or distract from the sense of professionalism within your practice site.

Distracting Nonverbal Communication

One of the most distracting nonverbal elements is lack of eye contact. It is frustrating to talk to somebody who is not looking at you. Unfortunately, many pharmacists unconsciously do not look at patients when talking to them. Their tendency is to look at the prescription, the prescription container, the computer screen, or other objects while talking. This behavior may indicate to patients that you are not totally confident about what you are saying or that you really do not care about speaking with them. Not looking at the patient also limits your ability to assess whether the patient understands the information. In other words, lack of eye contact limits your ability to receive feedback from the patient about the messages that you are giving. For instance, does the patient have a questioning look, an expression of surprise, or an expression of contentment and understanding? As discussed in Chapter 5, good eye contact is also essential for effective listening. If you do not look at patients while they are talking, they may get the impression that you are not interested in what they are saying. Using good eye contact does not mean that you continually stare at patients, because that may make them feel uncomfortable as well. The key is that you spend most of the time looking at them (see Figure 3-1).

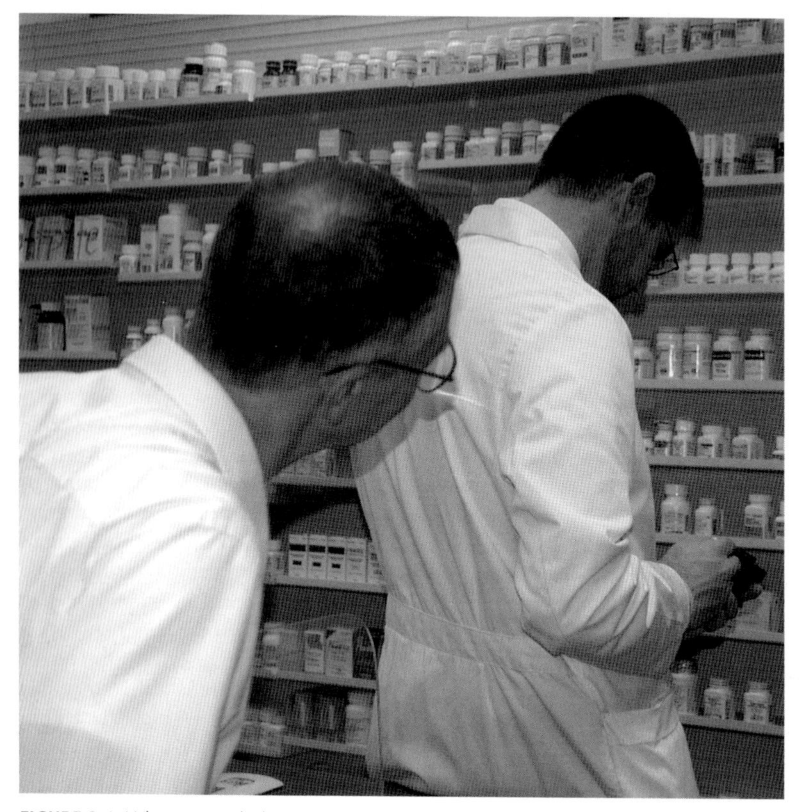

FIGURE 3-1. What nonverbal messages is the pharmacist sending? The patient?

Another potentially distracting nonverbal element is facial expression. An inadvertent facial expression may send a message that you did not intend to transmit. For example, if you roll your eyes as a patient explains something to you, you may be communicating a feeling of disinterest or lack of concern toward the patient. This is especially damaging when your facial expressions are not consistent with your verbal expressions. For example, if you say, "Go ahead, I am listening. Tell me about it!" but your eyes are distracted by something else in the pharmacy, you may be communicating mixed messages. The patient hears you say that you are interested, but your nonverbal behavior communicates otherwise. In these situations, people would tend to believe your facial expression and other nonverbal messages more than the verbal aspects of your communication.

In addition to facial expression, body position can be somewhat distracting. Most patients will judge your willingness to talk to them based on their perception of your body position. For example, a closed stance with folded arms or a body position that is slouched forward or tilted to one side may be communicating reluctance on your part to talk with them. You must be aware of your body position. Does it project your sincere desire to talk with your patients or does it show a lack of concern or interest?

Another potential distraction to communication may be your tone of voice. People interpret the message not only by the words you use, but also by the tone of voice you use. For example, a comment in a sarcastic or threatening tone of voice will produce a different effect than the same phrase spoken with an empathic tone. In addition, conveying a message in a dull, monotone voice may convey a lack of interest on your part. An inappropriate tone of voice may create an entirely different meaning from the one intended. To identify possible barriers, it may be useful to record yourself during interactions with your patients (with their permission) to reveal possible inconsistencies. You may find that you sound much different than you expected. You may think that you are communicating in an empathetic manner, but the recording may prove otherwise.

Detecting Nonverbal Cues in Others

Up to this point, this chapter has focused on your own nonverbal communication. The following section examines nonverbal messages provided by others and describes how to better detect these messages. Assessing the meaning behind the nonverbal messages of others is difficult, because we tend to interpret nonverbal cues based on our own personal backgrounds and experiences. We "filter" these messages based on our personal orientation and experiences. The meaning of the nonverbal message that we receive may or may not be the meaning intended by the sender. For example, we may sense a hint of anger in a patient's voice when in actuality the patient is using his or her normal speaking voice and the patient is not angry at all. The key is to identify situations where we might be misinterpreting their nonverbal cues based on these differences. We need to avoid making false assumptions or jumping to conclusions based on inaccurate interpretations of nonverbal cues. It would be impossible to list all the potential situations where differences could arise; however, we will focus on some of the most common issues.

The Importance of Nonverbal Communication in Health Care Encounters

For a patient, the illness experience can produce profound feelings of vulnerability and dependence. These emotions are often conveyed primarily through nonverbal channels. Pharmacists too experience emotions in providing care to patients, especially to those who are facing a serious illness. Research in medical care indicates that openness of emotional expressiveness on the part of health care professionals, including nonverbal indications of interest in the patient, is associated with greater patient satisfaction (Hall et al., 1995; Griffith et al., 2003). In addition, sensitivity on the part of providers to nonverbal patient cues has led to enhanced patient–provider relationships (Hall et al., 2009).

Some elderly and physically ill persons may have limited or impaired sense capabilities that will influence how they communicate nonverbally. Case Study 3.1 illustrates this point.

CASE STUDY 3.1

During his first externship experience in a community pharmacy, a pharmacy student (John) was assigned the task of receiving new prescriptions from patients. John wanted to help the patients and was looking forward to the opportunity of talking with them about their problems. One day, Mr. Stevens approached the prescription counter to have his prescription for levodopa refilled. John, who did not realize that Mr. Stevens had Parkinson's disease, noticed that his hands were shaking and commented, "I see you are a bit nervous today, Mr. Stevens. What's the matter?"

John observed a nonverbal message (rapid hand movement) from Mr. Stevens and assigned a wrong (and embarrassing) meaning to it. John should not have jumped to the conclusion based on just one nonverbal cue but should have noticed that Mr. Stevens' head was also moving and that he walked with a shuffled gait, which are other characteristics of Parkinson's disease.

This example illustrates that we need to adjust our communication in accordance with the messages that nonverbal cues are sending us. Another example occurs when elderly patients move closer to you or put a hand to their ears. What message might these nonverbal cues indicate? Possibly, they may indicate that they are having difficulty in hearing. You may also observe hearing aids, glasses, and other devices that indicate possible communication difficulties.

Another example occurs when patients are reluctant to speak to pharmacists and we do not know the real reason behind this behavior. Could it be a lack of respect for the pharmacist? Or could it be embarrassment? It is interesting to note that a Harris Survey (1997) found that embarrassment was the most common reason why consumers did not approach their health care provider. A wide variety of embarrassing issues could exist within practice, including incontinence, sexual dysfunction, depression, menopause, hemorrhoids, contraception, and breast or prostate cancer. As a pharmacist, you should be prepared to recognize situations that may be sensitive areas for patients. You should be comfortable discussing such matters in a nonthreatening way and in an environment that conveys confidentiality and privacy. Here are some tips and tactics to help with sensitive situations.

Watch your patients. Before engaging in a conversation, watch their behavior to get a clue about their feelings. They may appear to be embarrassed before they reach the prescription counter.

Discuss sensitive issues with clarity and avoid potentially frightening scenarios. For example, you may bring up the subject of incontinence by saying, "Miss Smith, would you like to step away to a quieter area so that we can talk?... Now, we have many women who get their prescriptions from us here for bladder control problems. While this problem is potentially embarrassing, there are several effective means to deal with it."

Be cognizant of the potential for nonadherence. Many patients with sensitive issues do not follow their medical regimens as directed. Check medication refill rates and observe patient behavior when they are describing how they take their medications. If you suspect nonadherence to medication regimens, ask open-ended questions to assess patient attitudes and feelings. For example, you could ask, "How do you feel about taking this medication?" This gives you an opportunity to watch and listen to both verbal and nonverbal messages.

Overcoming Distracting Nonverbal Factors

As mentioned earlier, the first step in improving interpersonal communication is recognizing how you communicate with others. In the nonverbal area, this self-awareness involves being constantly aware of your nonverbal behavior. In this regard, videotaping yourself is particularly helpful, since it reveals the positive and negative aspects of your nonverbal communication.

Once you have discovered what aspects you need to change to become more effective, the next step is a difficult one: finding strategies to overcome these distracting elements. Several suggestions have been already made to improve specific nonverbal elements. One thing that should be mentioned here is that potentially distracting behaviors can be overcome by using nonverbal elements that project different messages. For example, you may find that you naturally cross your arms while talking to others. You can overcome the possible perception that you are acting defensively by using other nonverbal elements, such as smiling, using a friendly tone of voice, or moving closer to the patient. The total message received by the patient is the combination of all these nonverbal cues, both positive and negative, and not just one isolated component. Another example is that if you have a soft voice and you sense that the patient cannot hear you, then you should lean toward the patient, raise your voice, or move the patient into a quieter section of the pharmacy. The key to this process is to first recognize distracting nonverbal elements and then try to overcome them.

Summary

Because nonverbal communication contributes significantly to the meanings of messages between pharmacists and others, it is important for you to keep the following in mind:

1. Certain nonverbal behaviors are universal; however, many are culturally specific.
2. Interpreting body language is ambiguous. Many people state that they can read a person like a book. However, assigning a particular meaning to a specific body movement without checking the meaning of that movement is dangerous. You could assign the wrong meaning to the nonverbal message.
3. Nonverbal behavior is more powerful than verbal. If the spoken word contradicts nonverbal behaviors, the observer will believe the nonverbal messages. Even simple advice, such as "Store this in the refrigerator and shake it well

every time you use it," may be influenced by your facial expression and tone of voice (Burgoon et al., 1995). If your tone conveys boredom and your manner is perfunctory, the advice may be seen as being of only minor importance.

4. The physical attributes of your practice environment have important effects on communication with patients. The location, design elements of the counseling area, employee appearance, and even the color scheme and signage on the walls all contribute to the messages that patients receive about your philosophy and attitude toward patient counseling.

Nonverbal communication involves an enormously important part of interpersonal communication. You should concentrate on your own nonverbal communications, as well as the various nonverbal cues provided by others. In this way, you can become a more effective, skilled communicator. Developing an awareness of your own nonverbal messages and detecting the nonverbal messages in others are important steps in developing skilled nonverbal communication. As discussed in Chapter 2, the communication process involves the transmission of both nonverbal and verbal messages in an environment plagued with barriers. An initial step in improving the communication process is to become more aware of these barriers.

REVIEW QUESTIONS

1. **How much communication is attributed to its nonverbal component? Why is this so?**
2. **What is the importance of cue clusters?**
3. **List the many ways that body language can improve your role as a pharmacist.**
4. **Differentiate between kinesics and proxemics.**
5. **Examine your own nonverbal behavior and list ways you may overcome any distracting styles.**

REVIEW CASES

REVIEW CASE STUDY 3.1

Mary Jane Marvel is a 22-year-old college senior. For the past semester, she has had what she perceived to be a nagging vaginal infection. She went to the Student Health Center and received a diagnosis of gonorrhea. She was so embarrassed and upset that she really didn't talk to the nurse practitioner about her treatment. She approaches the campus health pharmacy with trepidation and stands off to one side while Stephanie, the pharmacist, fills her prescription. Stephanie notices Mary Jane's behavior and leaves the prescription counter to talk with her.

REVIEW CASE STUDY 3.1, cont.

Stephanie: Hello, Miss Marvel, I am Stephanie Gonzales, and as the pharmacist who filled your prescription, I would like to talk to you a little bit about it. But before we talk, let's step over here to a more private area. Is this okay?

Mary Jane: Sure, why not (*said nervously*).

Stephanie: I was watching you a moment ago and you seem very distressed.

Mary Jane: How would you feel if you had *this disease*? Besides, why should I confide in you?

Stephanie: I can appreciate how you might feel, but I may be able to help by providing information about your treatment.

Mary Jane: Well, I guess I have to talk with someone ... I do want to discuss the medicine.

Stephanie: I respect your trust.

Mary Jane: I've got gonorrhea and I am scared I won't be able to have sex for a long, long time.

1. Discuss the various nonverbal messages that Mary Jane was sending.
2. Analyze Stephanie's ability to notice Mary Jane's nonverbal behavior.
3. Describe the environmental and emotional barriers that Stephanie needed to overcome in order to speak effectively with Mary Jane.
4. What nonverbal behavior could Stephanie display that indicates she is ready to listen and talk with Mary Jane?

REFERENCES

Borman EG, Nichols RG, Howell WS, Shapiro GL. *Interpersonal Communication in the Modern Organization*. Englewood Cliffs, NJ: Prentice-Hall, 1969.

Burgoon JK, Buller DB, Woodall WG. *Nonverbal Communication: The Unspoken Dialogue* (2nd ed., pp. 251–255). New York, NY: McGraw-Hill, 1995.

Griffith CH, Wilson JF, Langer S, Haist SA. House staff nonverbal communication skills and standardized patient satisfaction. *Journal of General Internal Medicine* 18:170–4, 2003.

Hall JA, Harrigan JA, Rosenthal R. Nonverbal behavior in clinician-patient interaction. *Applied & Preventive Psychology* 4:21–37, 1995.

Hall JA, Roter DL, Blanch DC, Frankel RM. Nonverbal sensitivity in medical students: Implications for clinical interactions. *Journal of General Internal Medicine* 24(11):1217–22, 2009.

Harris L. *Physician Patient Barriers to Communication*. National Harris Survey, 1997.

Keltner JW. *Interpersonal Communication*. Belmont, CA: Wadsworth, 1970.

Mehrabian A. *Silent Messages*. Belmont, CA: Wadsworth, 1971.

Poytos F. *New Perspectives in Nonverbal Communication*. New York, NY: Pergamon Press, 1983.

CHAPTER

4

Barriers to Communication

Overview

Within the communication process, numerous barriers exist that may disrupt or even eliminate interpersonal interaction. Given the large number of potential barriers that exist in pharmacy practice settings, it is a wonder that any communication takes place at all. Some barriers are rather obvious, while others are more subtle. The key is to identify when barriers exist and then develop strategies to minimize them. This chapter provides an overview of general barrier issues within communication and provides examples in a few key areas, such as practice environments, personal issues, administrative priorities, and lack of time and resources. Additional types of barriers are discussed in subsequent chapters as they relate to the more specific aspects of the communication process.

Introduction

Nothing could be more frustrating than to realize that you are not communicating effectively with another person. For example, you want to complain to your car mechanic that your car still does not run right. While you are telling him about your problem, the mechanic continues to look at a pile of papers on the counter and to mutter an occasional "uh-huh." You continue to relate in the best way you can the nature and urgency of your problem. However, he rushes over to the phone, papers in hand, and starts talking into the receiver without even looking up. While on the phone, he winks at you and says, "Go ahead, I'm still listening. Keep telling me about your problem." How do you feel—frustrated, angry, confused? Why? Probably because you feel you can't communicate with this person. He is not listening to you even though he says he is. Even if you have never experienced this specific situation, you can probably understand the frustration, anger, and confusion resulting from this lack of effective communication.

As indicated in Chapter 2, the communication process involves five essential elements: the sender, the message, the receiver, feedback, and barriers. Deficiencies in any of these essential elements may cause a breakdown in communication. The message must be clearly sent by the sender and received accurately by the receiver. Feedback that verifies understanding must be related in a clear, unambiguous manner. The fifth element, barriers, is often overlooked. Unfortunately, many things seem to get in the way when you try to communicate with someone else. Some issues are rather obvious, while others are not. Some barriers are easily removed, while others are more complex and require multiple strategies to minimize their impact.

Minimizing communication barriers typically requires a two-stage process: first, you must be aware that they exist. Second, you need to take appropriate action to overcome them. To become a more effective communicator, it is essential that you realize when you are not communicating effectively with another person and then try to analyze why effective communication is not taking place. This chapter focuses on some of the more common communication problems in pharmacy practice in the areas of environment, personal issues, administrative policies and procedures, and lack of time. Suggested strategies for minimizing their impact are also provided.

Environmental Barriers

The environment in which communication takes place is critical in pharmacy practice, and distractions within the environment often interfere with this process. Some environmental barriers are rather obvious, while others are more subtle. For example, in many community practice settings, glass partitions separate patients from pharmacy personnel. Although these partitions provide a private area for staff to work, they unfortunately may intimidate some patients and inhibit communication between patients and pharmacy staff. This type of environment may also give patients the impression that pharmacy staff do not want to talk to them. Ideally, the environment should provide areas where staff and patients can communicate face to face without physical barriers. This will also help counteract patient perceptions that pharmacy staff members are not approachable.

Crowded, noisy prescription areas also inhibit one-to-one communication in many practice settings. Many pharmacies have significant background noise, such as people talking or music playing. These noises interfere with your ability to communicate with patients. In addition, other people may be within hearing range of your conversation, which limits the level of perceived privacy for the

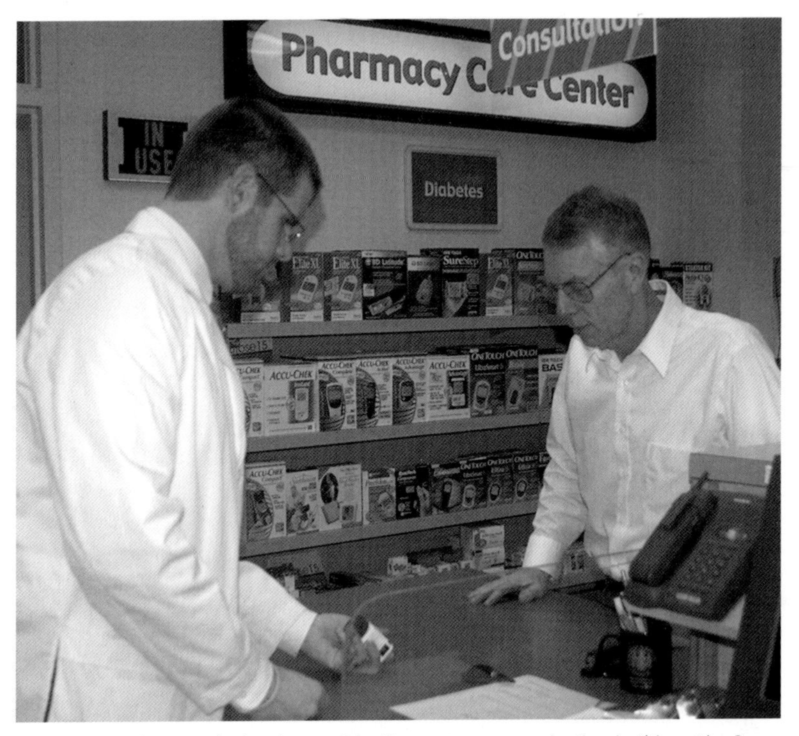

FIGURE 4-1. What are the barriers and facilitators to communication in this setting?

interaction. Privacy is especially important when patients want to talk about personal matters. Noise also interferes with your ability to use the phone effectively when trying to communicate with physicians, patients, and others.

Many community practitioners have tried to address these issues by increasing the amount of privacy with planters or room dividers to create the feeling of a private conversation area that is away from common traffic areas. Some have installed private or semiprivate counseling areas or rooms. Privacy does not necessarily mean having a private room, but both the patient and pharmacist must feel that privacy exists. Even in a busy, noisy environment, privacy can be enhanced by moving to the end of the prescription counter or by turning away from a busy prescription area and lowering your voice to achieve a more private environment.

Privacy issues also exist in institutional and ambulatory care clinics. Finding private locations to have meaningful discussions with nurses, physicians, or other health care practitioners can be problematic in many settings. For example, noisy hallways inhibit effective one-to-one interactions with your health care colleagues. Such encounters should not be heard by others due to the sensitive nature of these discussions and the high levels of professional ethics that most health care providers have. Thus, these conversations should take place in relatively private environments (Figure 4-2).

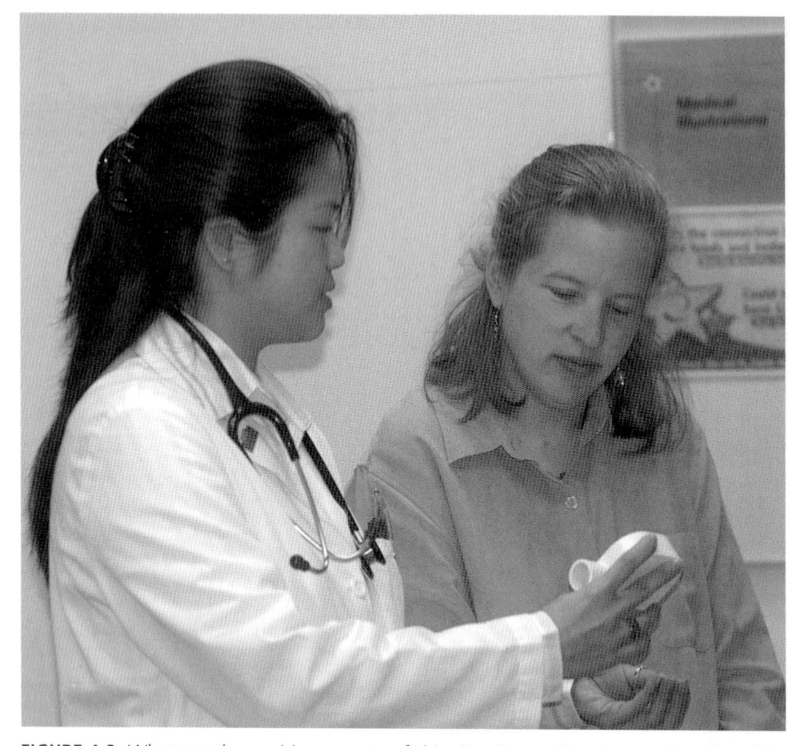

FIGURE 4-2. What are the positive aspects of this situation as the pharmacist talks with the patient in an ambulatory care clinic?

The first step in removing environmental barriers is discovering which of them exist in your practice setting. One approach might be to view things from the other person's perspective. What images do others have when they enter your practice site? How easy is it for them to access you to have a meaningful dialogue? How many steps does it take you to reach a private area within your practice site? (See Box 4.1 for other possible observations.) Paying attention to the amount of privacy can help create an atmosphere that causes both parties to communicate more effectively.

Within institutional practice, it may be helpful to observe where most interactions with physicians and nurses occur and what potential barriers may exist in these settings. For example, when nursing personnel visit in-patient pharmacies, typically they must interact with pharmacy personnel via a French-type door or a glass window. Unfortunately, the conversations of both parties can be heard by anyone working in the pharmacy or standing in the hallway. This is not the best setting for meaningful discussions about patient care issues or medication delivery issues. In busy patient care areas within institutions, you need to find ways to discuss patient-specific issues with your colleagues out of hearing range of family

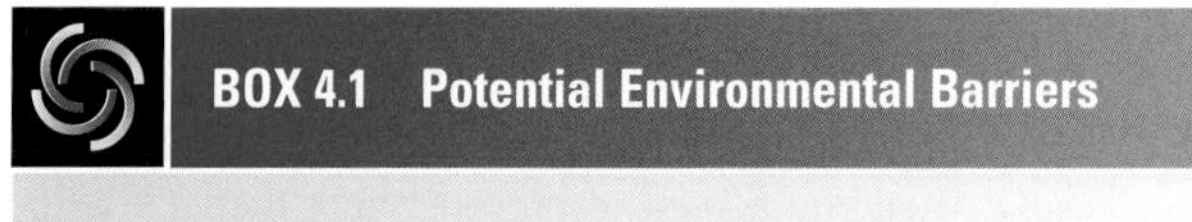

BOX 4.1 Potential Environmental Barriers

The next time you enter a community pharmacy, check for the following:

- Is the pharmacist visible?
- Is it easy to get the pharmacist's attention?
- Does it appear that the pharmacist wants to talk to patients?
- Is the prescription area conducive to private conversation?
- Do you have to speak to the pharmacist through a third party?
- Is there a lot of background noise or other distractions?

members, patients, and other individuals who happen to be in the area. When discussing therapy at a patient's bedside, you will need to be sensitive to patient needs as well. Most institutions, especially teaching institutions, have developed protocols and standards for how to engage in bedside conversation, recognizing the need to discuss clinical information and yet afford common courtesy toward the patient.

Personal Barriers

Many personal characteristics can lead to distractions in communication (see Box 4.2). Lack of confidence in your personal ability to communicate effectively may influence how you communicate. If you believe that you do not have the ability to communicate well or are rather shy, you may avoid talking with others. Many people feel that an effective communication style is something you are born with and may use this perception as an excuse to avoid interacting with others. Unfortunately, people do not realize that communication skills can be learned and barriers overcome. However, like other skills, they require practice and reinforcement. Positive reinforcement is critical since many times you may experience negative reinforcement in your attempts to communicate.

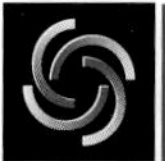

BOX 4.2 Potential Pharmacist-Related Personal Barriers

- Low self-confidence
- Shyness
- Dysfunctional internal monologue
- Lack of objectivity
- Cultural differences
- Discomfort in sensitive situations
- Negative perceptions about the value of patient interaction

For example, what might happen if you get into a heated argument with a patient who appears to be unreasonable and rude? Would you be excited to talk to the next patient? Probably not. What might happen if you felt you were taken advantage of by a colleague when you agreed to do something that you really didn't want to do? Would you feel like avoiding this individual in the future? Probably. These negative experiences may influence your personal desire to communicate and your self-esteem regarding interactions with others. As with most situations, future performance is based on past experiences—if you have had positive experiences in the past, you will probably be more confident when facing future encounters. You must remember that there are no expert communicators: No one communicates perfectly 100% of the time, and you should not be discouraged when it does not go as well as planned. However, you must still strive to improve your communication skills by constant practice and reflection on your strengths and weaknesses.

PHARMACIST-RELATED PERSONAL BARRIERS

A personal barrier for some pharmacists involves the degree of personal shyness. Individuals with high levels of shyness tend to avoid interpersonal communication in most situations, including interactions with patients, physicians, or other health care providers. These individuals have a high level of anxiety associated with communication with others. Many people feel that personal shyness is culturally based or may be linked to the inability to speak a second language. However, as noted by professionals working in this area, it goes beyond cultural issues and affects many native-born individuals as well. Overcoming this barrier requires time, effort, and, many times, professional assistance. Resolving personal shyness is a more complex process than overcoming other types of communication barriers. Techniques, such as systematic desensitization or cognitive modification, have been successful in resolving personal shyness for some persons (Baldwin et al., 1982). Since these strategies are far too complex to warrant further discussion in this text, we refer you to the counseling psychology literature for a broader discussion of possible strategies.

Another personal barrier to communication is the internal conversation you may have within yourself while talking with others. For example, while you are listening to someone, you may be thinking to yourself about how you want to deal with this situation. You might be thinking, "What in the world is she talking about?", "How can I get rid of this person?", or "I'm too busy to deal with her right now." This internal conversation may limit your ability to listen effectively as you focus on your own thoughts rather than on what the other person is saying. Often these internal conversations result in prejudging others or coming to a hasty conclusion about the perceived problem and suggested solutions. Internal messages are essential, because they allow you to sort things out while you are communicating. However, they become distracting if allowed to take precedence over what the person is actually communicating. It is difficult to recognize when you are more preoccupied with your own thoughts than with listening to the other person. It is essential to become aware of this habit because it can inhibit your ability to listen and can make you appear to be disinterested and rude.

Another potential personal barrier involves emotional objectivity. While taking care of patients, you may be tempted to take on their emotional problems. Many patients whom you will serve have multiple, complex problems, and you may be enticed to help them resolve emotional as well as physical issues. Although physical and emotional issues are often related to each other, you should separate your role in treating both. It may be appropriate for you to assist with physical issues, but probably not patient emotional needs. You should remain empathetic towards your patients, but not get so involved that you carry their emotional burdens with you. It is probably more appropriate to refer patients to professionals who can assist them with these issues.

Culturally based factors may also serve as personal barriers to effective communication. For example, in some cultures it is not proper to engage in eye contact during communication. Such behavior would be labeled as disrespectful, while in other cultures, direct eye contact is appropriate and is almost required. Other barriers related to culture include the following:

- Definitions of illness (some patients may not perceive themselves to be ill)
- Perceptions of what to do when ill (some cultures stress self-reliance rather than seeking help)
- Health-related habits or customs (eating habits)
- Health-seeking behavior (some cultures place more reliance on folk medicine)
- Perceptions of health care providers (based on possible distrust of the health care system or past negative experiences)

It is important to recognize that these and other cultural barriers may exist in the patients whom you serve.

Other personal barriers exist in situations where you may not be completely sure how to respond. For example, you may not know exactly what to say when a cancer patient expresses a fear of dying. Or, you may feel awkward when you need to talk to your superior about a sticky personnel problem at work. These personal fears or anxieties may put tremendous pressure on you to "say the right thing" and cause you to avoid interacting with others. Experience has shown that many times people tend to blow these types of situations out of proportion, making issues larger and more difficult than they really are; once they overcome their anxiety and eventually interact with others, the situations often turn out better than expected.

Another personal barrier involves the pharmacist's personal perception of the value of patient communication. Many pharmacists believe that talking with patients is not a high-priority activity. They may perceive that patients neither expect nor want to talk with them. Thus, they are reluctant to approach patients. If they do not value patient interaction, they will not be eager to participate in patient counseling activities. Unlike environmental barriers, removal of these barriers involves personal introspection and analysis of your motivation and desire to communicate.

PATIENT-RELATED PERSONAL BARRIERS

Several personal barriers relate to patients. For example, patient perceptions of pharmacists and pharmacy staff are critical in establishing communication rapport. If patients perceive you as not being knowledgeable or trustworthy, they will tend not to ask questions or listen to the advice being offered. Also, if they perceive that you do not want to talk with them, they will not approach you. On the other hand, if patients perceive you as being knowledgeable and have had positive experiences in the past, they will tend to seek out information. Therefore, you may need to alter negative patient perceptions by informing patients that you sincerely want to communicate with them and by actually counseling them effectively.

Another patient perception that hinders communication is their belief that the health care system is impersonal. Some patients sense that health care providers are not concerned about them as individuals but rather as cases or disease states. They may have been treated poorly in the past and may perceive you to be part of this impersonal system. Thus, you should assess the nature of your practice setting and the manner in which the pharmacy staff treats patients to make sure that you are not contributing to this impersonal atmosphere. If patients have positive feelings toward your environment, they will be more willing to talk with you and your staff.

Patient perceptions of their medical conditions may also inhibit communication. Some may believe that their condition is a relatively minor one requiring no further discussion with you. Thus, they may not seek out information from you, or they may rebuff your attempts to counsel them. In contrast, some patients may be overly anxious about their condition and therefore will avoid talking about it because they feel so vulnerable. Some patients may feel that their physicians would have already told them all the important information about their condition and their medication. Therefore, there is no need to talk with you. In addition, many patients think that all the important information is stated on the prescription label or in the patient education leaflet. You may need to convince some patients that they need to learn more about their medications and that the few moments spent with you will be valuable to them later on.

Administrative Barriers

Several factors dealing with the administrative aspects of pharmacy practice serve as barriers to communication. For example, most community practitioners are not paid directly for educating or communicating with patients. Counseling services are not included as part of pharmacies' business plans. Therefore, many pharmacy managers perceive the task of talking with patients as an expensive service and not a high priority. However, studies have shown that many consumers are willing to pay for such services (Suh, 2000). In addition, numerous initiatives have begun to document the costs and benefits of patient counseling in an effort to have pharmacists reimbursed by governmental programs and third-party insurance companies for this valuable service. Community pharmacists are being encouraged by professional organizations to seek reimbursement for the patient care services they provide.

Unfortunately, pharmacies often make policies that discourage pharmacist–patient interaction. Evidence of these policies is reflected in how certain community practice settings are organized and how they function. Policies related to the design of practice settings may deter counseling. In addition, the mechanics of dispensing prescriptions may distract from the communication process. It is difficult to complete all the necessary dispensing tasks while trying to communicate with the patient. Another subtle barrier is the pharmacist's desire to answer every phone call, which may give the impression to the patient that the pharmacist does not want to talk to him or her. Review case 4.1 illustrates how distractions could cause potentially harmful situations.

Staffing policies may also inhibit patient counseling. Many pharmacies have reduced the number of staff members who can assist pharmacists. Sufficient staff support should provide more time for the pharmacist to offer enhanced patient care, including patient counseling. In addition, work flow issues need to be monitored. Often, when patients need to talk with the pharmacist, they must first mention it to the assistant, who then relays the message to the pharmacist. In some situations, the pharmacist then responds to the assistant (rather than directly to the patient), who then passes the answer on to the patient. Obviously, this is not the best method of communication, because both the question and answer can be misinterpreted by any of these three parties. Mechanisms that allow patients to have ready access to the pharmacist need to exist. Support staff needs to be aware of situations where patients need to talk with the pharmacist. Training of staff is a crucial component to enhancing patient care. Review case 4.1 describes an actual pharmacy practice experience resulting from a breakdown in administrative policies, which resulted in the assistant and the pharmacist not double-checking the name of the intended patient or checking the patient's identity when the prescription was picked up.

Time Barriers

Choosing an inappropriate time to initiate conversation may lead to communication failure. The timing of the interaction is critical, since both parties must be ready to communicate at a given time. For example, a woman who just came from a physician's office after waiting for 3 hours with two sick children may not be interested in talking with you or anyone else. The most important thing on her mind is to go home, get her kids to bed, and then relax. She is probably not in the best frame of mind to sit down and have a meaningful conversation about her children's medications. Another example might be when a mother is too busy texting a message to her husband while she is receiving instructions about her child's medication. She is not really paying attention to anything around her. Another is when you try to speak to a physician who is running between appointments and perceives your phone call as an intrusion into his practice.

By the same token, you may not be in the best frame of mind to interact with others. You may be dealing with multiple issues: a physician is waiting on the phone, a large number of prescriptions need to be filled in the next hour, and you have not eaten lunch so you are starving. You may feel that this is not a convenient time to talk to others, such as the mother in the above example. A possible solution might be to give the mother basic information to get the therapy started and then contact her at a later time via phone or e-mail when both of you may be more relaxed and ready to communicate. Another strategy is to have written information that can reinforce a short message during busy situations. Many pharmacists make efficient use of time during these brief counseling encounters by "highlighting" pertinent information within the written information to emphasize key points before the patient leaves the pharmacy.

Timing within institutional practice is also critical, since health care providers are performing multiple tasks in very active environments. It may be difficult to get people's attention and to choose the right time to interact with each other. Many times there is a sense of urgency, since there is no assurance that you will see the physician, nurse, or other health care provider later in the day due to their busy schedules, so you need to find the best way to tactfully approach them.

Summary

Interpersonal communication, because of its complexity and human involvement, is a fragile process. Messages become helpful to others only when they are accurately received and understood. If messages are distorted or are incorrect, they actually may be harmful to patient care and interpersonal relationships. Failure to communicate may lead to negative patient outcomes. Barriers, such as the ones discussed in this chapter, may lead to distortion of messages and misunderstandings between you and others. As discussed in Chapter 6, you must be assertive about your need to communicate with others, but at the same time be aware of their needs as well. In any situation, you should assess nonverbal messages from health care providers or patients for assurances that communication is well timed (Do they appear to be listening to you? Are they comprehending what you are saying?). At the same time, you must be aware of situations where people are trying to talk with you, but you are not listening appropriately. It is important to recognize the potential barriers involving the environment, personal issues, administrative policies, and timing and then to develop strategies to minimize or remove them. Additional barriers are discussed in the remaining chapters as they relate to more specific aspects of the communication process.

REVIEW QUESTIONS

1. **What is the first step in removing environmental and personal barriers to communication?**
2. **What are at least three patient barriers that inhibit communication?**
3. **How can the current nature of pharmacy practice inhibit good communication?**

REVIEW CASES

REVIEW CASE STUDY 4.1

A pediatrician phoned two different antibiotic prescriptions into a pharmacy—one for Brian Bentley and one for Brandon Bentley. Unfortunately, the pharmacy assistant did not recognize that two different names were given and did not realize that they were twins. She subsequently typed both prescriptions for Brian (Brandon sounded like Brian to her). The father picked up both prescriptions and gave them both to Brian. Unfortunately, the parents did not discover the error until the next day. They immediately called the pharmacy to address the issue. Both the assistant and pharmacist on duty apologized to the Bentleys; fortunately, Brian was not injured by taking a few doses of both antibiotics.

1. Name three things that help facilitate communication in this setting.
2. Describe three things that help facilitate communication in this ambulatory care clinic.

REFERENCES

Baldwin HJ, Richmond VP, McCroskey JC, Berger BA. Quiet pharmacist. *American Pharmacy* NS22:24–27, 1982.

Suh DC. Consumers' willingness to pay for pharmacy services that reduce risk of medication related problems. *Journal of the American Pharmacists Association* 40:818–827,876–878, 2000.

CHAPTER

Listening and Empathic Responding 5

Overview

Listening to patients—trying to understand their thoughts and feelings—is crucial to effective communication. However, empathic communication requires more than understanding. The understanding you have must be conveyed back to patients so they realize that you *do* understand. In addition, you must genuinely care about patients and not be afraid to communicate your concern to them. Finally, patients' feelings must be accepted without judgment as to being "right" or "wrong." This chapter examines various skills involved in listening and empathic communication. The attitudes essential to empathic communication and the effects of such communication on pharmacist–patient relationships are also explored.

Listening Well

When we think about skills of "effective communication," we probably think first of the skills involved in speaking clearly and forcefully and in having an effect on others based on the persuasiveness of what we say. However, an equally critical part of the communication process, and perhaps the most difficult to learn, is the ability to be a good listener. You have probably experienced a sense of satisfaction and gratitude when you have felt that the other person really listened to what you had to say and, to a large extent, understood your meaning. In the relationship between a health professional and a patient, the patient's feeling of being understood is therapeutic in and of itself. It helps to ameliorate the sense of isolation and helplessness that often accompanies a patient's experience of illness as well as the frustration involved in negotiating the health care system. Your ability as a pharmacist to provide your patients with the sense that they are understood is a crucial part of your effectiveness in communicating with them.

Chapter 2 described the components of the interpersonal communication model and explained the importance of the feedback loop to effective communication. As the receiver of messages, your ability to listen well influences the accuracy with which you are able to decode messages in a way that is congruent with a patient's intended message. In addition, your ability to convey your understanding back to patients will affect the degree to which they feel understood and cared for. If you fail to understand the patient, this can be uncovered and clarified in the feedback process. If your attempt to listen and understand is genuine, even "missing the mark" will usually not be damaging if the overall message being conveyed is one of caring and acceptance.

In addition to the communication barriers discussed in previous chapters, some communication habits can interfere with your ability to listen well. Trying to do two things at once makes it evident to patients that they do not have your full attention. Planning ahead to what you will say next interferes with actively trying to understand the meaning of patients' communication. Jumping to conclusions before patients have completed their messages can lead to only hearing parts of messages—often pieces that fit into preconceived ideas you have. Focusing only on content, judging the person or the message as it is being conveyed, faking interest, and communicating in stereotyped ways all cause us to miss much of the meaning in the messages people send us. See Figure 5-1.

Listening well involves understanding both the content of the information being provided and the feelings being conveyed. Skills that are useful in effective listening include (1) summarizing, (2) paraphrasing, and (3) empathic responding. Empathic responding, as described below, includes "reflection of feeling" statements that verbally convey your understanding of the essence or emotional meaning of another person's communication. In addition, nonverbal communication that shows caring and attention to the patient is a crucial component of effective listening.

SUMMARIZING

When a patient is providing information, such as during a medication history interview, it is necessary for you to try to summarize the critical pieces of information. Summarizing allows you to verify that you understood accurately the information conveyed by the patient and allows the patient to add new information that may have been forgotten. Frequent summary statements serve to identify misunderstandings that may exist, especially when there are barriers in communication, such as language barriers.

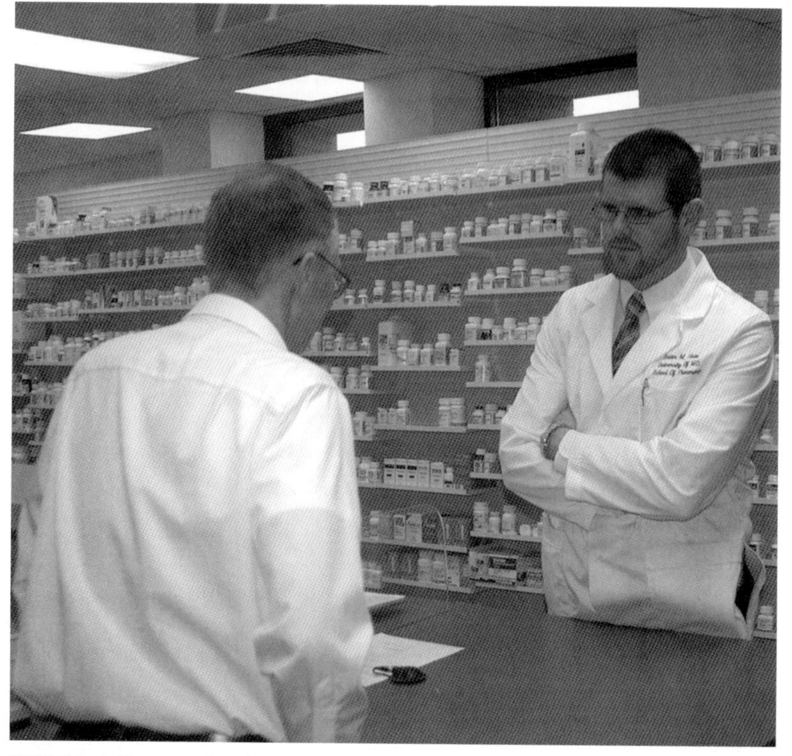

FIGURE 5-1. How can the pharmacist improve his attending behaviors?

PARAPHRASING

When using this technique, you attempt to convey back to the patient the essence of what he or she has just said. Paraphrasing condenses aspects of content as well as some superficial recognition of the patient's attitudes or feelings. The following are examples of paraphrasing:

Patient #1: I don't know about my doctor. One time I go to him and he's as nice as he can be. The next time he's so rude I swear I won't go back again.

Pharmacist #1: He seems to be very inconsistent.

Patient #2: I'm glad I moved into the retirement village. Every day there is something new to do. There are always lots of things going on—I'm never bored.

Pharmacist #2: So there are a lot of activities to choose from.

Empathic Responding

Many of the messages patients send to you involve the way they feel about their illnesses or life situations. If you are able to communicate back to a patient that you understand these feelings, then a caring, trusting relationship can be established. Communicating that you understand another person's feelings is a powerful way of establishing rapport and a necessary ingredient in any helping relationship.

THEORETICAL FOUNDATIONS

The importance of empathy in helping relationships has been elucidated most eloquently by psychologist Carl Rogers (Rogers, 1957, 1967). Rogers developed person-centered psychotherapy, which is part of a humanistic tradition in psychology. Central is the belief that, if individuals are able to express themselves honestly in an accepting, caring atmosphere, they will naturally make healthy decisions for themselves. In such an environment, people are able to reach solutions to their emotional problems that are right for them. Thus, pharmacists can be helpful by providing a "listening ear" to help patients clarify feelings. The ability to listen effectively to the emotional meaning in a patient's message is the essence of empathy. Rogers (1957) described empathy as follows:

> To sense the client's private world as if it were your own but without ever losing the 'as if' quality...To sense the client's anger, fear, or confusion as if it were your own, yet without your own anger, fear, or confusion getting bound up in it.

Rogers goes on to emphasize the necessity of both accurately understanding the client or patient and effectively conveying back to the patient, briefly and in your own words, what you understand his or her experience to be. Empathy conveys understanding in a caring, accepting, nonjudgmental way. Rogers (1967) has noted the lack of empathy in most of our communications:

> I suspect that each of us has discovered that this kind of understanding [empathy] is extremely rare...Instead, we offer another type of understanding which is very different, such as 'I understand what is wrong with you' or 'I understand what makes you act that way.'

The main difference between an empathic response and a paraphrase is that empathy serves primarily as a reflection of the patient's feelings rather than focusing on the content of the communication. The following examples, adapted from the section on paraphrasing, should illustrate the difference.

Patient #3: I don't know about my doctor. One time I go to him and he's as nice as he can be. The next time he's so rude I swear I won't go back again.

Pharmacist #3:

Paraphrase: He seems to be very inconsistent.

Empathic Response: You must feel uncomfortable going to see him if you never know what to expect.

Patient #4: I'm so glad I moved into the retirement village. Every day there is something new to do. There are always lots of things going on—I'm never bored.

Pharmacist #4:

Paraphrase: So there are a lot of activities to choose from.

Empathic Response: You seem to love living there.

In addition to using empathic responses, two other attitudes or messages must be conveyed to the patient if trust is to be established. First, you must be genuine, or sincere, in the relationship. If the patient perceives you as phony, your "caring" a well-practiced facade, then trust will not be established. Being genuine may mean, at times, setting limits in the relationship. For instance, it may be necessary to tell a patient that you do not have time right now to discuss an issue in detail, but will telephone or set an appointment for when you are not so busy. The fact that you were direct and honest about your limits will probably do less to harm the relationship than if you had said, "I'm listening," while nonverbally conveying hurry or impatience. The discrepancy between what we say and how we act sets up barriers that are difficult to overcome.

Another essential condition is respect for and acceptance of the patient as an autonomous, worthwhile person. If you convey an ongoing positive feeling for patients, they may be more open with you since they do not fear that they are being judged. They will be more likely to tell you they do not understand regimen directions if they know you will not think them "stupid." They will be more willing to reveal they are having trouble taking their medications as prescribed if they do not fear you will perceive them as being incompetent or careless. One of the biggest blocks to effective communication is our tendency to judge each other. If we think that another will judge us negatively, we feel less willing to reveal ourselves. Acceptance and warmth, if genuine, allow patients to feel free to be more open in their communication with you.

Although Carl Rogers died in 1987, research studies on what he described as the "core conditions" for a helping relationship have continued and have, in fact, increased in number since his death (Kirschenbaum and Jourdan, 2005). A meta-analysis (Greenberg et al., 2001) found a statistically and clinically significant relationship between empathy and positive therapeutic outcomes. The factor most related to positive outcome was the patient's perception of being understood. More recent conceptualizations of therapeutic relationships have described the "therapeutic alliance" between the provider and the patient, which includes the core condition of empathy (Orlinsky et al., 1994; Martin et al., 2000; Feller and Cattone, 2003). In addition, recent theories of how providers can facilitate health behavior change, including the Motivational Interviewing approach discussed in Chapter 8, describe empathy as a crucial element in the provider–patient relationship (Miller and Rollnick, 2002).

While Carl Rogers is most closely associated with describing empathy and its positive effects in therapeutic relationships, other branches of psychotherapy, including psychodynamic and cognitive–behavioral schools, have noted the essential nature of the provider's empathy in helping patients. Some theorists have focused on cognitive components of empathy and have viewed it as a stable trait that depends on an individual's underlying ability to take the differing perspectives of others (Hogan, 1969). Others have emphasized affective components and emotional responsiveness as central to empathy. Davis (1983, 2006) conceptualizes empathy as requiring both perspective taking and emotional responsiveness where an empathic person vicariously experiences the emotions of others. While acknowledging the cognitive and affective components, most of the work in medicine and pharmacy has focused on the communicative aspects of empathy and has thus emphasized the behavioral component, conceptualizing it as a skill that can be learned.

EMOTIONAL RESPONSES TO ILLNESS

Many of the messages patients send to providers involve the way they feel about their illnesses or those of loved ones. Feelings of fear, frustration, and vulnerability are an inevitable component of coping with illness. Patients want to know their fears and concerns are understood. The perception that feelings are understood by the health professionals they rely on is therapeutic in and of itself. Empathy helps patients come to trust you as someone who cares about their welfare. Your expression of caring and understanding can help to alleviate the patient's sense of isolation, which often accompanies an illness experience. Pharmacists may hesitate to respond to patients' expressions of emotions because "I'm not a psychologist." However, the fact that patients confided in you means they want you to know about their experiences. Failure to acknowledge or understand is, in fact, damaging to the relationship. Such a response conveys the impression that the pharmacist's role in health care does *not* include understanding patients' feelings about their illnesses or concerns about their treatment.

Empathy and Effective Communication

Empathy has many positive effects on a pharmacist's relationships with patients. It helps patients come to trust you as someone who cares about their welfare. It helps patients understand their own feelings more clearly. Often their concerns are only vaguely perceived until they begin to talk with someone. In addition, an empathic response facilitates the patient's own problem-solving ability. If they are allowed to express their feelings in a safe atmosphere, patients may begin to feel more in control by understanding their feelings better. Patients may also feel freer to explore possible solutions or different ways of coping with their own problems.

As an example, put yourself in the role of a community pharmacist. Your patient, Mr. Raymond, talks about his physician: "I've been to Dr. Johnson several times because I heard he was a good doctor. But he just doesn't seem to care. I have to wait endlessly in the waiting room even with an appointment. Then when I do get to see him, he rushes in and out so fast I don't have a chance to talk to him. Oh, he's pleasant enough. I just get the feeling he doesn't have time to talk to me." Which of the following comes closest to being the type of response you would find yourself making to Mr. Raymond? Place a "1" next to a statement that you would definitely use, place a "2" next to a statement that you might use, and place a "3" next to a statement that you would never use.

______ a. "You have to understand that Dr. Johnson is a very busy man. He probably doesn't mean to be abrupt."

______ b. "Dr. Johnson is a very good physician. I am sure he gives patients the best care possible."

______ c. "I don't blame you for being upset. You shouldn't have to wait that long when you have an appointment."

______ d. "Tell him how you feel about the way he treats patients. Otherwise, find a different physician."

______ e. "I'm sure you just happened to see him when he was having a bad day. I bet if you keep going to him, things will improve."

______ f. "I know how you feel. I hate to wait in doctors' offices, too."

______ g. "No one feels that they have enough time to talk with their doctors."

______ h. "How long do you usually have to wait before you get in to see him?"

______ i. "Let me talk with you about the new prescription you're getting."

______ j. "You seem to feel there's something missing in your relationship with Dr. Johnson—that there isn't the caring you would like."

Now that you have indicated which statements you are likely to give, it is important to analyze how Mr. Raymond may perceive each statement. Many times, we attempt to say something that we feel is valuable to patients, but our statements are perceived very differently by the patient. This is due, in part, to possible hidden messages that we convey. Consider the possible hidden messages that you may have conveyed to Mr. Raymond with each of the above responses.

JUDGING RESPONSE

While conveying understanding seems so obviously a part of good communication, a number of less helpful responses are frequently used in communication with others. Often, for example, we tend to judge or evaluate another's feelings. We tell patients in various ways that they "shouldn't" feel discouraged or frustrated, they "shouldn't" worry, and they "shouldn't" question their treatment by other health professionals. Any message from you that indicates you think patients are "wrong" or "bad" or that they "shouldn't" feel the way they do will indicate that it is not safe to confide in you. In the example above, responses [a] ("You have to understand that Dr. Johnson is a very busy man. He probably doesn't mean to be abrupt.") and [b] ("Dr. Johnson is a very good physician. I'm sure he gives patients the best care possible.") indicate that you thought Mr. Raymond was "wrong" or that he misperceived the situation. In either case, the judgment was conveyed that he "shouldn't" feel as he does. Even response [c] ("I don't blame you for being upset. You shouldn't have to wait that long when you have an appointment.") is an evaluative judgment that Mr. Raymond's feelings are "right" or "justified" and implies that it is appropriate for you to judge his feelings as "right" or "wrong."

ADVISING RESPONSE

We also tend to give advice. We get so caught up in our role as "expert" or "professional" that we lose sight of the limits of our expertise. Obviously, we must, as pharmacists, give patients advice on their medication regimens. That is part of our professional responsibility. However, the advising role may not be appropriate in helping a patient deal with emotional or personal problems. The best source of problem solution resides within the patient. It is presumptuous of us to feel we can offer a quick "solution" to another's personal concerns. In addition, it conveys to patients that we do not perceive them as competent to arrive at their own decisions. Even when the advice is reasonable, it is not a decision that patients have arrived at themselves. Relying on others for advice may keep patients "dependent," seeing others as the source of problem solving. In the example with Mr. Raymond, your advice in response [d] ("Tell him how you feel about the way he treats patients. Otherwise, find a different physician.") gives a quick (and rather presumptuous) "solution" to what is a complex problem in the eyes of Mr. Raymond.

There are times when patients do want advice and are looking for help with their problems. Assisting them in identifying sources of help they can call on may be an appropriate way to help patients. Suggesting alternatives for consideration may also be helpful. In this type of response, you are serving as a sounding board for decisions the patient makes rather than providing your own solutions.

There are times, of course, when patients are not capable of coping with their own feelings or problems. A typical example is the patient who is severely depressed. Being able to recognize the signs of depression and referring patients to sources of help, such as the family physician or a local mental health service, are professional functions you must be prepared to perform. However, most people who are ill have transient feelings of depression and worry that are typical reactions to illness. They need to be provided with concerned, empathic care.

PLACATING OR FALSELY REASSURING RESPONSE

A third mode of response to a patient's feelings is a placating or falsely reassuring response. Telling a patient who is facing surgery, "Don't worry, I'm sure your surgery will turn out just fine" may seem to be helpful, but is really conveying in a subtle way that the person "shouldn't" feel upset. We often use this kind of response to try to get a patient to stop feeling upset or to try to change a patient's feelings, rather than accepting the feelings as they exist. This type of response may be used even when the patient is facing a situation of real threat, such as a terminal illness. We may feel helpless in such a situation and use false reassurance to protect ourselves from the emotional involvement of listening and trying to understand the patient's feelings. Response [e] ("I'm sure you just happened to see him when he was having a bad day. I bet if you keep going to him, things will improve.") is a falsely reassuring response that predicts a positive outcome you have no way of knowing will occur.

GENERALIZING RESPONSE

Another way in which we try to reassure patients is by telling them, "I've been through the same thing and I've survived." While it is sometimes comforting to know that others have had similar experiences, this response may take the focus away from the patient's experience and onto your own experience before the patient has had a chance to talk over his or her own immediate concerns. It also can lead you to stop listening because you jump to the conclusion that, since you have had an experience similar to the patient's, the patient is feeling the same way you felt. This may not, of course, be true. Response [f] ("I know how you feel. I hate to wait in doctors' offices, too.") would fit in this category. Response [g] ("No one feels that they have enough time to talk with their doctors.") also indicates that Mr. Raymond's feelings are not unique or special in any way. The "everyone feels that way" response, again, is meant to make Mr. Raymond feel better about his problem, but instead makes him feel that you do not consider his concerns to be very unique or important.

QUIZZING OR PROBING RESPONSE

Another type of response to feelings is a quizzing or probing response. We feel comfortable asking patients questions—we have learned to do this in medication history taking and in consultations with patients on over-the-counter drugs. However, asking questions when the patient has expressed a feeling can take the focus away from the feeling and onto the "content" of the message. It also leads to the expectation that, if enough information is gathered, a solution will be forthcoming. Many human problems or emotional concerns are not so easily "solved." Often patients simply want to be able to express their feelings and know that we understand. Meeting those needs for a "listening ear" is an important part of the helping process. Asking Mr. Raymond how long he has to wait for an appointment (response [h]) does not convey an understanding of the essence of his concern, which was his perception of a lack of caring from his physician.

DISTRACTING RESPONSE

Many times we get out of situations we don't know how to respond to by simply changing the subject. With response [i] ("Let me talk with you about the new prescription you're getting.") Mr. Raymond gets no indication from you that his concerns have even been heard, let alone understood.

UNDERSTANDING RESPONSE

Contrast each of the other responses to Mr. Raymond with response [j]. ("You seem to feel there's something missing in your relationship with Dr. Johnson – that there isn't the caring you would like.") Only in this response is there any indication that you truly understand the basis of Mr. Raymond's concern. By using such a response, you convey understanding without judging Mr. Raymond as right or wrong, reasonable or unreasonable.

The above discussion reviewed different responses that you may make to feeling statements. The dialogue in Case Study 5.1 is an example of a patient–pharmacist communication that may invite quite different reactions from the patient. The situation involves Mrs. Raymond, who engages the pharmacist, Jeff Brown, in conversation when she picks up a prescription for her husband, George. The patient–pharmacist conversation is in the left column, and an analysis of the conversation is in the right column.

CASE STUDY 5.1

Initial Approach

Conversation	Analysis
Mrs. Raymond: (*deep sigh*) George has been sick for so long; sometimes I wonder if he's ever going to get well. I don't know if I can keep my spirits up much longer.	
Jeff: Now, of course George is going to get well and you can keep your spirits up. You've been so strong about it.	**Placating response:** Mrs. Raymond's reaction to this might be "How can he be so sure George will get well? And he thinks I've been so strong: He has no idea how terrified I've been most of the time."
Mrs. Raymond: But it's been so long. It seems that Dr. Johnson should be getting George well pretty soon.	Mrs. Raymond seems to be protesting Jeff's glib response that she has nothing to worry about.
Jeff: Now, you know Dr. Johnson is a good doctor and you shouldn't be questioning his care of your husband. It's important to trust your physician.	**Judging response:** Mrs. Raymond's response to this might be "Of course, he'd stick up for the physician. And it isn't really that I question his treatment of George. I'm just discouraged and no one understands that."
Mrs. Raymond: Well, he's certainly not getting anywhere with George!	
Jeff: How long has it been now that George has been sick?	**Quizzing or probing response:** Having this bit of information at this point is probably not as important as focusing on Mrs. Raymond's feelings.

Conversation	Analysis
Mrs. Raymond: Thirteen months.	
Jeff: Sometimes these things take time. Maybe you just need to get away more. I think it would do you good to have someone come in and stay with George, say one day a week, so you can get out more.	**Advising response:** While this advice may be reasonable, the fact that Jeff offered this as a quick solution may outrage Mrs. Raymond. It's as if he can presume to tell her how to cope with the situation when she has been coping with it for 13 months. If anything, she could probably teach him a thing or two about coping.
Mrs. Raymond: I don't want to get out more. I want George to get well.	
Jeff: He will, believe me. He is getting the best care possible.	

Contrast the above exchange with the following between Mrs. Raymond and Bill Reynolds, another pharmacist.

Second Approach

Conversation	Analysis
Mrs. Raymond: (*deep sigh*) George has been so sick for so long, sometimes I wonder if he's ever going to get well. I don't know if I can keep my spirits up much longer.	
Bill: It must be heartbreaking to see George so ill.	**Understanding response:** Bill shows that he recognizes the stress that Mrs. Raymond has been under.
Mrs. Raymond: It is. I sometimes feel that it's hopeless.	Mrs. Raymond confirms that Bill is accurate in his understanding and goes on to reveal a little more about her feelings.

Bill: You seem discouraged	
Mrs. Raymond: (*Head nod and nonverbal struggle to control tears*)	Often the response to an accurate understanding will not be further exploration of feelings. The fact that someone has listened and understood may be all she needs at the time. Bill lets her decide how much she wishes to reveal by leaving the door open without forcing disclosure through probing.
Bill: (*after long pause*) Is there something I can do to help?	
Mrs. Raymond: Sometimes it helps just to be able to talk to people. Dr. Johnson always tells me not to worry. How can I help but worry?	
Bill: It sounds as if people try to cheer you up instead of understanding how painful it is for you.	
Mrs. Raymond: I don't blame Dr. Johnson. I know he's a good doctor. But sometimes I get frustrated by how long it's taking.	

A patient who feels discouraged or angry often needs simply to know that others understand. Mrs. Raymond is not "blaming" Bill or the physician but is lashing out because of her own frustrations and feelings of helplessness. Rather than placating her ("He's getting the best care possible") or judging her feelings ("You shouldn't be questioning his [physician's] care of your husband"), the pharmacist can be helpful instead by showing concern and understanding.

We try in various ways to get patients to stop or change their feelings. We may feel uncomfortable in dealing with expressions of emotion, so, to protect ourselves, we cut off patients' communication of feelings. We may try to distract them by changing the subject; we may try to show them that things are not as bad as they seem; or we may direct the communication to subjects we feel comfortable with, such as medication regimens. These responses tend to convey to patients that we are not listening and, perhaps, that we do not *want* to listen. Yet it is a gratifying experience for a patient to feel that someone has listened and, to a large extent, understood the feelings expressed. As a pharmacist, monitoring how well you are listening to patients is as important as carefully choosing the words you use in educating them about their medications.

Attitudes Underlying Empathy

Underlying empathic responding is an empathic attitude toward others. This attitude means that you want to listen and try to understand a person's feelings and point of view. It means you are able to accept feelings as they exist without trying to change them, stop them, or judge them. You are not afraid of a patient's emotions and are able to just *be* with the person and not necessarily *do* anything except listen. An empathic person is able to trust that people can cope with their own feelings and problems. If this attitude is held, you will not be afraid to allow patients to express their feelings and arrive at their own decisions. An empathic person also believes that listening to someone is helpful in and of itself. In fact, it is often the only means of help you have to offer. Health professionals feel frustrated and helpless if they cannot prescribe a medication and "cure" a patient's problems. Yet the emotional concerns patients bring to you along with their physical problems cannot be "cured" or "treated" in that way. This does not mean that you have no help to provide; it does mean that you must define "helping" in a new way.

In addition, with empathic communication, it is not sufficient to feel that you understand another person—empathy requires that you effectively convey to the person that you do, in fact, understand. How can this be done? One approach is to briefly summarize what you understand the person's feelings to be. In the conversation between the second pharmacist (Bill) and Mrs. Raymond, Bill said, "You seem discouraged," which captured the essence of what Mrs. Raymond had been communicating and served to convey to her that Bill had heard and understood her concerns.

The ability to summarize the essence of a patient's feelings and convey this understanding back to the patient involves what is called "reflection of feeling." Reflection of feeling has been defined as restating in your own words the essential attitudes and feelings expressed by the patient. Reflection of feeling is not simply a repetition of what the patient has said; instead, it conveys your attempt to grasp the meaning of the patient's communication. It further implies that you are checking to make sure that your understanding is accurate. In this sense, the reflection of feeling is not a bold, declarative statement but rather a tentative and provisional one. For example, Mrs. Raymond describes another problem to Judy Lang, the pharmacist:

> My daughter seems to get sick a lot – headaches or nausea and vomiting. I've had her to the doctor but he says there's nothing wrong. I've noticed that she seems to get sick whenever there's a big exam she's supposed to take or a speech she's supposed to give at school. It isn't that I think she's faking, mind you. She really is sick – vomiting and everything.

If Judy were to respond "Your daughter seems to get sick a lot – usually right before a big exam at school," she is simply repeating what Mrs. Raymond has told her. Mrs. Raymond might reasonably respond, "That's what I just told you, isn't it?" However, if Judy were to go beyond the surface meaning of Mrs. Raymond's statement and try to reflect her concern in fresh words, Judy's response might be something like this: "It sounds like you're afraid your daughter may be reacting to the stress she feels at school by becoming physically ill. Is that what you think is happening?"

Judy's response captured Mrs. Raymond's concern but was put into Judy's own words and so was perceived by Mrs. Raymond as showing understanding.

In this response, Judy did not jump to unreasonable or unsupported conclusions about what the problem was. Her response is a tentative "Let's see if I understand" kind of response. In addition, she avoided any threatening labels or interpretations such as "You seem to feel your daughter's illnesses are psychosomatic." Such a word would have been too "clinical" and frightening for Mrs. Raymond and would have hindered Judy's attempt to show understanding.

If Judy had tried to convey her understanding by saying, "I know how you feel" or "I understand your concern," the response would not have been as effective as a reflection of feeling response in conveying empathy. "I understand" is a cliché that can be used as a standard response to any feeling statement and thus is not perceived as a response unique to the person with whom you are talking. Because the response also does nothing to convey *what* your understanding is, it is much less personal and effective than actually trying to reflect the feeling the patient is expressing.

An empathic response implies neither agreement nor disagreement with the perceptions of the patient. If a patient says to you as manager of a pharmacy, "Your clerk was extremely rude to me. She acts as if she doesn't care about your customers," your first impulse may be to check up on the facts. While this is, of course, important and necessary, it does not convey understanding of the patient's perceptions. The patient talking to you does not *feel* cared for, regardless of what the objective truth about the clerk's behavior happens to be.

EMPATHY CAN BE LEARNED

There is a widespread belief that empathic communication skills are not something one can learn. The belief is based on the notion that you either are an empathic person or you are not. As with any new behavior, learning to alter existing habits of responding *is* very difficult. Pharmacists who are not accustomed to conveying their understanding of the meaning of illness and treatment for their patients will at first feel awkward using empathic responses. As with any new skill, being an empathic listener must be practiced before it becomes a natural part of how we relate to others. However, empathic communication skills can be learned if pharmacists have value systems that place importance on establishing helping relationships with patients. As health care providers, we must develop communication skills that allow us to effectively convey our understanding and caring to patients.

EMPATHY AND TRUST IN HEALTH PROFESSIONAL–PATIENT RELATIONSHIPS

The trust patients have in their health care providers means they have confidence that providers will act in their best interests. Mechanic and Meyer (2000) describe the vulnerability of patients and the risks they take in trusting people they hardly know (health professionals) in circumstances where misplaced trust can have devastating consequences. These investigators identified interpersonal (not technical) competence as the principal component mentioned by patients as key to trust in their providers. The traits identified most often were the provider's willingness to listen and the provider's ability to display caring, concern, and compassion. In addition to helping establish trust in patient–provider relationships, the provider's recognition of, and problem-solving response to, the patient's emotional distress has been found to be related to actual reduction in the patient's emotional distress (Roter et al., 1995).

Nonverbal Aspects of Empathy

In conveying your willingness to listen, your nonverbal behavior is at least as important as what you say. As discussed earlier, you can do a number of things nonverbally to convey your interest and concern. Establishing eye contact while talking to patients, leaning toward them slightly with no physical barriers between you, and having a relaxed posture all help to put the patient at ease and show your concern. Head nods and encouragements to talk are also part of empathic communication. A tone of voice that conveys that you are trying to understand the person's feelings also complements the verbal message. Establishing a sense of privacy by coming out from behind the counter and getting away from others who may be waiting help convey your respect for the patient. Conveying that you have time to listen—that you aren't hurried or distracted—makes your concern seem genuine.

Sensitivity to patients' nonverbal cues is also a necessary part of effective communication. Asking yourself "How is this person feeling?" during the course of a conversation will lead to the discovery that feelings and attitudes are often conveyed most dramatically (sometimes exclusively) through nonverbal channels. A person's tone of voice, facial expression, and body posture all convey messages about feelings. To be empathic, you must "hear" these messages as well as the words patients use.

Problems in Establishing Helping Relationships

There are countless sources of problems in interpersonal communication between pharmacists and patients. However, certain pharmacist attitudes and behaviors are particularly damaging in establishing helping relationships with patients. These include stereotyping, depersonalizing, and controlling behaviors. The following section describes these common deficiencies and offers suggestions for improvement in these key areas.

STEREOTYPING

Communication problems may exist because of negative stereotypes held by health care practitioners that affect the quality of their communication. What image comes to mind when you think of an elderly patient?...a patient on welfare?...a chronic pain patient?...a noncompliant patient?...an illiterate patient?...a "hypochondriacal" patient?...a dying patient?...a "psychiatric" patient? Even the label "patient" may create artificial or false expectations of how an individual might behave. If you hold certain stereotypes of patients, you may fail to listen without judgment. In addition, information that confirms the stereotype may be perceived while information that fails to confirm it is *not* perceived. For example, if a pharmacist has a negative stereotype of people who use analgesics, especially opioids, on a chronic basis, he may view a patient who complains about lack of effective pain control as "drug seeking" rather than as someone who is not receiving appropriate and effective drug therapy.

What does the issue of stereotyping mean for pharmacists? First, before we can be effective in communicating with patients, we must come to know what stereotypes we hold and how these may affect the care we give our patients. We must then begin to see our patients as individuals with the vast array of individual differences that exist. Only then can we begin to relate to each patient as a person, unique and distinct from all others.

DEPERSONALIZING

Unfortunately, there are a number of ways communication with a patient can become depersonalized. If an elderly person is accompanied by an adult child, for example, we may direct the communication to the child and talk about the patient rather than with the patient. We may also focus communication on "problems" and "cases." Many aspects of disease management make communication narrow and impersonal. For example, discussing only the disease or the problems a patient might have managing treatment without commenting on the successes in treatment or even the everyday aspects of the patient's life places the focus on narrow clinical rather than broader personal issues. A rigid communication format of a pharmacist monologue rather than pharmacist–patient dialogue can also make communication seem rote and defeat the underlying purpose of the encounter.

CONTROLLING

Numerous studies have found that an individual's sense of control is related to health and feelings of well-being (Rodin, 1968; Langer, 1983; Taylor et al., 2000). A review of literature (Taylor et al., 2000) concluded that beliefs such as perceived personal control and optimism actually protect both the mental and physical health of individuals. When health care providers do things that reduce the patient's sense of control over decisions that are made regarding treatment, they may actually be reducing the effectiveness of the therapies they prescribe. Fostering a sense of control in patients is important in patient–practitioner relationships (see Schorr and Rodin, 1982, for a description of the theoretical foundation). Interventions to increase levels of patient participation and control in the provider–patient relationship have yielded positive results that include improved clinical and quality-of-life outcomes (Kaplan et al., 1989).

Yet actual communication between health care providers and patients may decrease rather than enhance the perceived personal control of the patient (Schorr and Rodin, 1982). Illness often results in disturbing feelings of helplessness and dependence on health care providers. Added to this patient vulnerability is the unequal power in relationships between providers and patients and the tendency of providers to adopt an "authoritarian" style of communicating. Patients are "told" what they should do and what they should not do—decisions are made, often with very little input from the patient on preferences, desires, or concerns about treatment. Yet in the process of carrying out treatment plans, patients do make decisions about their regimens—decisions of which we may remain unaware. In this way, patients reassert control of the management of their own conditions.

Labeling certain patient decisions as "nonadherence" is not helpful. Such labeling misses the point that the goal of treatment is to help patients improve health and well-being; it is *not* to get them to do as they are told. Instead of blaming the patient, we must appreciate the degree to which treatment decisions are inevitably shared decisions. We must ensure that information and feedback are conveyed by both patients and ourselves in a give-and-take process. We must actively encourage patients to ask questions and urge them to discuss problems they perceive with treatment, complaints they have about their therapy, or frustrations they feel with progress. This encouragement requires above all else our empathic acceptance of the patient's feelings and perceptions. Patient input is not seen as peripheral to the provision of health care. Instead, we see the patient as the center of the healing process. Establishing a relationship where patients are active participants in making treatment decisions and in assessing treatment effects is crucial to provision of quality care.

Knowing When to Refer

Responding with empathy to the concerns that typically accompany illness is the responsibility of all providers. However, dialogue with a patient may reveal that there are underlying problems that require more in-depth counseling or medical treatment. For example, a patient may reveal that they are under a lot of stress at work and want to buy an OTC sleep aid to help with their sleep problems. Your open communication with them may lead you to suspect there is an underlying depression that requires professional counseling or a medical referral. Another example may be a patient who is recently bereaved and, while the difficulty coping is a normal part of grieving, may require more extensive communication with a person trained in helping to cope with loss. A crucial skill in responding to a patient's emotional concern is knowing how to identify when a person needs help that you are not able to provide, knowing sources of referral in the community (preferably knowing specific persons that you can identify by name who can provide assistance), and being able to communicate in a caring way that there are others who are capable of helping more than you are. The message to the patient is, thus, that you understand the pain they are experiencing, that you want to help, but that you really don't have the training to provide the help they need in coping with their current situation. In some cases, the patient may be able to identify someone they would feel comfortable confiding in, such as their minister. Even referral to their primary care provider can be a first step in helping them get appropriate treatment.

REVIEW QUESTIONS

1. **Describe the four skills of effective listening, that is, summarizing, paraphrasing, empathic responding, and nonverbal attending.**
2. **Empathic responding has several positive effects. What are they?**
3. **How can active listening be inhibited by stereotyping, depersonalizing, and controlling?**

Summary

Listening well is not a passive process; it takes involvement and effort. It also takes practice to be able to convey understanding in a way that makes it seem natural rather than mechanical or artificial. However, when a relationship between you and a patient is marked by empathic understanding, the patient is helped in ways medications cannot touch.

REFERENCES

Davis MH. Measuring individual differences in empathy: Evidence for a multidimensional approach. *Journal of Personality and Social Psychology* 44:113–126, 1983.

Davis MH. Empathy. In Stets J, Turner J (eds.). *The Handbook of the Sociology of Emotions*. New York: Springer Press, 2006.

Feller C, Cattone RR. The importance of empathy in the therapeutic alliance. *Journal of Humanistic Counseling, Education and Development* 42:53–61, 2003.

Greenberg LS, Elliott R, Watson JC, Bohart AC. Empathy. *Psychotherapy* 38:380–384, 2001.

Hogan R. Development of an empathy scale. *Journal of Consulting and Clinical Psychology* 33: 307–316, 1969.

Kaplan SH, Greenfield S, Ware JE Jr. Assessing the effects of physician-patient interactions on the outcomes of chronic disease. *Medical Care* 27:5110–5127, 1989.

Kirschenbaum H, Jourdan A. The current status of Carl Rogers and the person-centered approach. *Psychotherapy: Theory, Research, Practice, Training* 42:37–51, 2005.

Langer EJ. *The Psychology of Control*. Beverly Hills, CA: Sage, 1983.

Martin DJ, Garske JP, Davis MK. Relation of the therapeutic alliance with outcome and other variables: A meta-analytic review. *Journal of Consulting and Clinical Psychology* 68:438–450, 2000.

Mechanic D, Meyer S. Concepts of trust among patients with serious illness. *Social Science and Medicine* 51:657–668, 2000.

Miller W, Rollnick S. *Motivational Interviewing: Preparing People for Change* (2nd ed.). New York, NY: Guilford Press, 2002.

Orlinsky DE, Grawe K, Parks BK. Process and outcome in psychotherapy. In Garfield SL, Bergin AE (eds.). *Handbook of Psychotherapy and Behavior Change* (4th ed., pp. 270–376). New York: Wiley, 1994.

Rodin J. Aging and health: Effects of the sense of control. *Science* 233:1271–1276, 1986.

Rogers CR. The necessary and sufficient conditions of therapeutic personality change. *Journal of Consulting and Clinical Psychology* 21:95–103, 1957.

Rogers CR. The therapeutic relationship: recent theory and research. In Patterson CH (ed.). *The Counselor in the School*. New York: McGraw Hill, 1967.

Roter DL, Hall JA, Kern DE, et al. Improving physicians' interviewing skills and reducing patients' emotional distress: A randomized clinical trial. *Archives of Internal Medicine* 155:1877–1884, 1995.

Schorr D, Rodin J. The role of perceived control in practitioner-patient relationships. In Wills TA (ed.). *Basic Processes in Helping Relationships*. New York: Academic Press, 1982.

Taylor SE, Kemeny ME, Reed GM, et al. Psychological resources, positive illusions, and health. *American Psychologist* 55:99–109, 2000.

CHAPTER 6

Assertiveness

Overview

Assertive pharmacists take an active role in patient care. These pharmacists initiate communication with patients rather than wait to be asked questions. Assertive pharmacists also convey their views on the management of patient drug therapy to other health care professionals. Finally, assertive pharmacists try to resolve conflicts with others in a direct manner but in a way that conveys respect for others.

Beginning Exercise

Before reading further, stop and ask yourself these questions:

1. If a group in your community asked you to give a speech on medication use, how would you respond?
2. When a patient is hostile, how do you tend to respond?
3. How many patients and physicians you talk with know you by name?
4. How often do you make it a point to talk with patients getting new prescriptions to make sure they understand their therapy? How often do you counsel only if they ask questions?

5. How frequently do you look at profile records and ask patients questions during refill visits to make sure medications are being taken appropriately, that therapeutic goals are being met, and that there are no problems with therapy?

The questions posed may seem to deal with diverse, unrelated situations—giving speeches, coping with criticism, and counseling patients. Yet they all involve situations where you can choose to act assertively or nonassertively.

Defining Assertiveness

What is assertiveness? Assertiveness is perhaps best understood by comparing it with two other response styles: passivity and aggression. These three styles of responding are described below.

PASSIVE BEHAVIOR

This response is designed to avoid conflict at all cost. Passive or nonassertive persons will not say what they really think out of fear that others may not agree. Passive individuals "hide" from people and wait for others to initiate conversation. They put the needs or wants of other people above their own. They tend to have a great deal of anxiety in relationships. They worry about how others will respond to them and have a high need for approval. Problems arise when people who behave passively feel secretly angry or resentful toward others. Passive persons may see themselves as victims who are subject to the manipulation of others. It is this view that is damaging to their self-esteem.

AGGRESSIVE BEHAVIOR

Aggressive people seek to "win" in conflict situations by dominating or intimidating others. Aggressive persons promote their own interests or points of view but are indifferent or hostile to the feelings, thoughts, or needs of others. Often, aggression seems to work as others back down in order to avoid prolonging or escalating the conflict. Because aggressive behavior may have beneficial effects in the short term, individuals may be reluctant to give up aggressive strategies. Often people who turn to aggression to reach their goals have a distorted view such that they constantly perceive themselves to be in threatening situations, to be under personal attack, or to be plagued by others trying to thwart their efforts. Such individuals are easily angered and have a low tolerance for frustration. They seem to believe that they should not have to experience frustration. Rather than the rational experience of disappointment, the aggressive person responds with indignant anger. Rather than helping to resolve problems, "getting it off your chest" usually serves to escalate the anger and aggression.

While others may give in to the intimidation of aggressive individuals initially, they can also act in subtle ways to "get even." For example, patients who do not feel they are treated with respect in a community pharmacy may not return to that pharmacy and may tell friends about their negative experiences. Employees who feel helpless and undervalued can sabotage the goals of their employer in a variety of indirect ways. Thus, aggressive individuals may "win" certain interpersonal battles in the short term, but their behavior often leads to negative long-term consequences.

Unfortunately, many aspects of our culture (media, television, movies, and politicians) reinforce the notion that the way you get your way is by using aggressive behaviors. You push your personal agenda without regard to other individuals' perspectives. Although people may achieve their own personal objectives using aggressive approaches, these strategies do not build trusting relationships, which is a key element in working with patients and others in professional practice. Thus, to be more effective in the long run, you must learn how to focus your energies using assertive, not aggressive, behaviors.

ASSERTIVE BEHAVIOR

Assertive behavior is the direct expression of ideas, opinions, and desires. The intent of assertive behavior is to communicate in an atmosphere of trust. Conflicts that arise are faced and solutions of mutual accord are sought. Assertive individuals initiate communication in a way that conveys their concern and respect for others. The goal of communication is to stand up for oneself and to solve interpersonal problems in ways that do not damage relationships. Assertiveness requires that you respect others as well as yourself.

Conflict is inevitable in human relationships. While conflict is usually viewed as undesirable, the process of resolving conflict can lead to growth and increased understanding and respect for others, in spite of differences. Problems arise when conflict leads us to view others as "opponents," when power differences are exploited, or when problem-solving discussions become unfocused with side issues brought in to derail the conversation.

A critical factor in being assertive is the ability to act in ways that are consistent with the standards we have for our own behavior. When we tell ourselves that other people "make" us feel or act a certain way, we are not taking responsibility for our own behavior. Instead of changing ourselves, we try (impotently) to get others to change. We believe that, as Mark Twain noted, "Nothing so needs reform as other people's habits." However, the only power we have to effect change in any relationship is to change our own behavior. For example, you may wish that your boss, who tends to be very negative during annual performance evaluations of staff, was more supportive of your work. However, just hoping that she would be more positive in her evaluations will not resolve this issue. You must take active steps to change how you respond to her criticisms rather than waiting for her to change her approach.

Too often, our goals in communication are defined in terms of what we want others to do rather than what we will do. For example, we might say that we want physicians to appreciate the role of the pharmacist in patient care. Redefining this goal would have us focus on what specific things we can do to improve our working relationships with physicians. If we tell others our goals in providing pharmaceutical care services and show them by our behavior what we want to achieve, many will come to respect our position. However, even if we fail to convince a physician that the role we play in patient care is of value, it does not mean we have failed in reaching the goals we have set for our own communication. When our goals focus on what we will do, we have control over our ability to meet these goals.

Research has shown that a number of skills are needed for assertive communication. These include initiating and maintaining conversations, encouraging assertiveness in others, responding appropriately to criticism, giving negative feedback acceptably, expressing appreciation or pleasure, making requests, setting limits or refusing requests, conveying confidence both verbally and nonverbally, and expressing opinions and feelings appropriately. Several of these strategies are described in a section on assertiveness techniques later in this chapter.

Theoretical Foundations

Assertiveness training and theories about how people learn to respond in passive or aggressive ways grow primarily out of cognitive and behaviorist psychological theories. Behaviorists believe that passive or aggressive responses have been reinforced or rewarded and thus strengthened. Aggressive behavior often works in the short term because others feel intimidated and allow aggressive persons to get what they want. Passive behaviors are reinforced when individuals are able to escape or even avoid conflict in relationships and thus escape the anxiety that surrounds these conflicts. Cognitive theories hold that people respond passively or aggressively because they have irrational beliefs that interfere with assertiveness. These beliefs involve

1. Fear of rejection or anger from others and need for approval (everyone should like me and approve of what I do)
2. Overconcern for the needs and rights of others (I should always try to help others and be nice to them)
3. Belief that problems with assertiveness are due to unalterable personality characteristics and are, therefore, unchangeable (this is just how I am)
4. Perfectionist standards. (I must be perfectly competent. If I am not, then I am a failure. Others must also be perfectly competent and deserve to be severely criticized if they are not.)

Because these beliefs are excessively perfectionistic, they are considered irrational. In the passive person, they create anxiety that leads the individual to try (unsuccessfully) to avoid the inevitable conflicts that arise in relationships. These unrealistic standards are also turned on others, leading to angry, aggressive behavior, with frequent "blaming" of others for their normal human failings. Cognitive restructuring, an assertiveness technique, teaches people to identify self-defeating thoughts that produce anxiety or inappropriate anger in difficult situations and replace them with more reasonable thoughts. As these new thoughts replace the self-defeating thoughts, they begin to be incorporated into the person's belief system. For example, as a pharmacist you may feel "used" by a boss who always counts on you for emergency coverage. You might currently say to yourself, "I don't want to come in to work on my day off this week, but if I say 'no' the boss will get mad, and that would be awful." Because this causes you anxiety at the imagined catastrophic consequences of saying "no," your response is inhibited. A more rational thought process when faced with such a request would be "I don't want to work on my day off this week. It is my right to say no. I am not responsible for solving all the problems my manager has in finding backup coverage." This thought reduces anxiety and frees you to practice new, more assertive responses to difficult situations.

Assertiveness Techniques

There are a number of communication techniques or strategies that are useful in responding to situations that tend to be conflict-ridden.

PROVIDING FEEDBACK

Letting others know how you respond to their behavior can help to avoid misunderstandings and also help to resolve the conflicts that are inevitable in relationships. However, providing honest feedback when you have a negative reaction to another person's behavior is difficult to accomplish without hurt feelings. Many times, you must tell people that you are upset by what they did in order to improve your relationship in the long run. When you choose to convey negative feedback to others, use techniques to make the communication less threatening. Criteria for useful feedback include the following:

- Feedback focuses on a person's behavior rather than personality. By focusing on behavior, you are directing the feedback to something the individual can change.
- Feedback is descriptive rather than evaluative. Describing what was said or done is less threatening than judging why you assume it was done.
- Feedback focuses on your own reactions rather than the other person's intentions. Assigning "blame" or assuming malevolent intent behind the behavior is not part of constructive feedback.
- Feedback uses "I" statements that take the form "When you [do or say] _____, I feel ___." For example, "When you are late for work, I feel frustrated and angry" is less damaging than "You're irresponsible. You don't care about the patients who are waiting and the coworkers covering for you when you're late."
- Feedback is specific rather than general. It focuses on behavior that has just occurred and avoids dragging in past behavior. It also does not overgeneralize from the specific instance that has upset you (e.g., "you always do ___").
- Feedback focuses on problem solving. The intent is not to let off steam. The intent is to solve a problem in a relationship so that the relationship can be improved.
- Feedback is provided in a private setting.

INVITING FEEDBACK FROM OTHERS

As mentioned above, we need to work on providing feedback in an appropriate manner. At the same time, we need to invite feedback from others in order to improve our interpersonal communication skills. For example, as a pharmacist, you should routinely assess patient satisfaction and invite feedback on your services. As a manager, you should let employees know that you welcome suggestions from them on how to improve pharmacy operations. Your ability to hear criticism or suggestions without defensiveness or anger, to admit when you have made a mistake, and to encourage feedback from others (even when it is negative) encourage people to be honest in their communications with you. These responses also allow you to identify areas of your professional practice that may need improvement and help to promote better relationships with others.

SETTING LIMITS

For some of us, setting limits on how we will spend our personal time and money is a source of frustration. We have difficulty saying "no" to any request. As a result, we feel overwhelmed and, often, angry at others for "taking advantage" of us. Being assertive in setting limits means that you take responsibility for the decisions you make on how to spend personal resources without feeling resentful toward others for making requests. Being assertive in setting limits does not mean that you stop saying "yes" to requests. You will no doubt continue to help others, even though doing so may be an inconvenience, because of the value system you hold and your desire to help others when they need help.

When faced with a request, the first step is to decide how much you are willing to do in meeting the request. If you need time to decide, delaying a response is appropriate as long as you get back to the person within the time frame you specify. Often a response may not be "yes" or "no" but an offer to partially meet the request. Saying "no" or setting limits may be particularly difficult if you believe that the other person must agree that you have a good reason for saying "no." If feelings of guilt trap you, you may not want to provide specific reasons for your decisions. In any case, you have the right to make the decision on how you will spend personal time and financial resources.

MAKING REQUESTS

Asking for what you want from others in a direct manner is also necessary in healthy relationships. If you are in a management position, clearly communicating your expectations of others is an important part of carrying out the goals of the organization. In equal relationships, making requests, including asking for help, is an important part of honest communication. We must trust that others will be able to respond to our requests in an assertive manner, including saying "no." Thus, we must not overreact when someone turns down our request in an assertive way.

BEING PERSISTENT

One important aspect of being assertive is to be persistent in assuring that your rights are respected. Often when you have set limits or said "no," people will try to coax you into changing your mind. If you continue to repeat your decision calmly, you can be assertive without becoming aggressive and without giving in. This response of calmly repeating your decision is often called the "broken record" response (Smith, 1975). It will stop even the most manipulative person without assigning blame or escalating the conflict.

REFRAMING

Frames are "cognitive shortcuts that people use to help make sense of complex information" (Kaufman et al., 2003). Reframing techniques described by Kaufman and colleagues include the following:

- Focus on developing effective communication around a set of limited objectives.
- Examine the potential validity of the other person's perspectives.
- Establish a common ground. Search for areas of agreement and focus on desired outcomes with a long-term perspective.
- Identify opportunities to explore solutions not yet pursued and opportunities for "trade-offs" or compromises.
- Finally, identify differences that cannot be bridged and at the same time explore conflict reduction actions that can still be taken.

IGNORING PROVOCATIONS

Interpersonal conflict may elicit various ways of trying to "win" by attempting to humiliate or intimidate others. For example, patients who are angry or feeling helpless may lash out with personal attacks. Pharmacists who feel unfairly criticized may respond in an aggressive or sarcastic manner. Interpersonal conflicts between health professionals are often marked by struggles for power and autonomy (often called "turf battles"). Ignoring the critical comments of others and focusing exclusively on solving underlying problems can do much to keep conflict from escalating to the point that relationships are damaged.

RESPONDING TO CRITICISM

For some of us, criticism is particularly devastating because we typically hold two common irrational beliefs: (1) that we must be loved or approved of by virtually everyone we know and (2) that we must be completely competent in everything we do and never make mistakes. Since such perfectionist standards are impossible to achieve, we are constantly faced with feelings of failure or unworthiness. In some cases, we may even have a desire to "get even" by launching into a counterattack on the person levying the criticism. The only way to counteract such feelings and cope reasonably with criticism is to begin to challenge the underlying, irrational beliefs that lead us to fear the disapproval of others.

How do assertiveness problems relate to your ability to function more effectively as a pharmacist? Let's examine a few typical situations in pharmacy practice and determine what might be the most assertive way to respond in relationships with patients, physicians, employees, employers, and colleagues.

Assertiveness and Patients

Perhaps the most important assertive skill in relating to patients is your willingness to initiate communication. Certain activities distinguish assertive pharmacists from passive ones. For example, some pharmacists seem to hide behind the counter, give prescriptions to clerks to hand to patients, and generally avoid interaction with patients unless asked specific questions. In this way, passive pharmacists are able to avoid the potential conflicts inherent in dealing with people and are able to hide their own feelings of insecurity and fears about being incompetent. While a passive approach may arise out of (or at least be rationalized by) a feeling of time pressure, passive pharmacists make no attempt to find alternative ways of providing better patient care, such as giving patients well-developed medication leaflets and calling them during slower hours to discuss key points and assess problems. Instead, passive pharmacists deal with things as they come and take the path of least resistance in providing minimal levels of pharmacy services. In contrast, assertive pharmacists come out from behind counters, introduce themselves to patients, provide information on medications, and assess the patient's use of medications and problems with therapy.

Encouraging patients to be more assertive is also an important skill in improving your communication with them. Helping patients prepare for visits with health professionals and encouraging their active participation in consultations have been found to improve communication and make patients more assertive in asking questions (Roter, 1977, 1984; Kaplan et al., 1989; Kimberlin et al., 2001). When asked to provide feedback about problems with medication therapy or errors in care, both hospitalized (Weingart et al., 2005) and ambulatory (Gandhi et al., 2003) patients could identify adverse events regarding treatment that would have remained unrecognized if they had not pointed them out.

You as a pharmacist may encourage patients to be more assertive by suggesting that they keep a list of questions about their therapy that they want to ask during their next visit. You may also have patients fill out brief questionnaires when they arrive at the pharmacy in which they write down their questions or concerns about their health or treatment. You could even give them a short checklist of informational items or issues about medications and ask them to check those items they would like to discuss with you. This process can help patients organize their thoughts and can counteract the passivity patients may adopt in the presence of a health professional. During their visits, you can actively solicit questions, concerns, and preferences regarding health care. Even normally assertive patients may experience enough anxiety in communication with providers that they forget to ask questions or bring up concerns they have.

A particularly difficult situation that you will face in pharmacy practice is responding to an angry or critical patient. While no one likes to hear criticism, there are ways of dealing with criticism in a rational, assertive manner. When you hear criticism from patients, it is important to keep in mind that their feelings of hostility may be greatly magnified by the life stresses they are experiencing. Patients are usually ill, sometimes seriously ill, and may be feeling helpless and dependent on health professionals. They may feel shuffled about, kept waiting in physician offices, and finally kept waiting for a prescription. It is important, therefore, to keep in mind that some (do not assume all) patient anger arises from frustrations about being ill, and not from personal grievances against you.

When patients are reacting primarily to the stresses of being ill, it is most helpful for you to understand what it is like for them and to respond empathically. An empathic response when patients react with shock and dismay at the cost of their medications will probably be more helpful than an attempt to justify the cost. Saying, "You're right. These medications are expensive. Are you worried about whether you can afford them?" shows that you understand the patient's worry and allows you to assess whether the concern about cost is a real problem of inability to afford treatment or a way of expressing diverse feelings of frustration.

Another skill that is useful in responding to patient criticism is to get patients to turn criticism into useful feedback. For example, if a patient tells you that your pharmacy does not seem to care about the customer, it is important to find out specifically what is causing the problem. Asking "What specifically is it that upsets you?" may give you feedback that would be useful in improving your pharmacy operation. You now have the information you need in order to decide whether you should make changes to improve patient care. Alternatively, you may decide to continue with current policies, but might see the need to better communicate your reasons for these decisions to patients.

There will be times with angry patients where you will need to stand up for yourself. If a patient persists in aggressive behavior in spite of your efforts to focus on understanding and problem solving, you will want to set limits without becoming aggressive. You can calmly tell an angry patient "I want to hear your point of view, but I do not want to be called names. When you are ready to talk without yelling and swearing, I will listen."

Assertiveness and Other Health Care Professionals

When problems in patient medication therapies arise, consultations with physicians or nurses are often required. If you have determined that you need to speak directly with the prescribing physician, you will be most effective if you are persistent with receptionists and nurses in your request. Messages transmitted through third parties may not be the most effective means of communication. Such persistence might sound something like the conversation in Case Study 6.1.

The pharmacist in this communication was assertive. He showed respect for the nurse and yet was persistent in stating his request. He did not argue about the issue of which method of communication was quicker. He calmly restated his request without anger or apology. Now, let's say you have managed to get through to the physician. Compare the following introductory comments by a pharmacist:

CASE STUDY 6.1

Pharmacist calling a physician's office: This is John Landers, the pharmacist at Central Pharmacy. I'd like to speak to Dr. Stone, please.

Nurse: He's with a patient right now. What is it you wish to speak to him about?

Pharmacist: I am concerned about Mrs. Raymond's prescription for metformin. I will need to speak to Dr. Stone about it. Please have him call me as soon as he comes out from the patient examination.

Nurse: It might be quicker if you tell me what the problem is. I could talk to Dr. Stone and get back to you.

Pharmacist: Thank you, but in this case I would like to talk to Dr. Stone directly.

Nurse: He's very busy today, and we're running behind schedule.

Pharmacist: I know he has a busy schedule, but I must speak with him as soon as possible. Please ask him to call.

a. Dr. Stone, this is the pharmacist at Main Street Pharmacy. I'm sorry to bother you—I know you're busy—but I think there's a problem with Mrs. Raymond's prescription for metformin.
b. Dr. Stone, this is John Landers, the pharmacist at Main Street Pharmacy. I'm calling about a problem Mrs. Raymond is having with her prescription for metformin.

In [a], the pharmacist did not introduce himself, which makes him an anonymous employee of a pharmacy rather than a professional with an individual identity. Also, in [a], he subtly "apologizes" for calling, which makes him seem insecure and unassertive.

Here are several ways the pharmacist could proceed:

a. Did you know that Mrs. Raymond is still having diarrhea from the metformin? Do you want to change her prescription?
b. I spoke with Mrs. Raymond today. She reports that she continues to have diarrhea after 3 months on the medication. She has stopped her walking program and is reluctant to leave the house because of the diarrhea. The effect on her life is so serious that you may want to consider switching her to a sulfonylurea such as glyburide, which is less likely to cause diarrhea.

Response [b] is better. The pharmacist is not putting the physician on the spot by asking him if he knew there was a problem. Instead, he presented the problem that concerned him and suggested alternative medications that could possibly resolve the problem.

When identifying potential problems, you should be prepared to identify alternatives to try to resolve the problem and to make your own recommendation on the preferred alternative. In order to do this with confidence, you should have checked references before making the phone call or sending the written communication. Having information on current research and citing it to convince the physician will increase your effectiveness in making a recommendation. Once you are sure of your facts, it is easier to be persistent in pushing for a therapeutic change that is required. Be sure that you feel prepared to use the medical terms and speak to the physician as a fellow health professional. Focus on the goal you share with the physician, which is to help the patient. When changes in therapy are agreed upon, it should be clear how the changes will be implemented (e.g., who will inform the patient) and what the monitoring plan will be to verify that the patient's problem has been resolved.

You are faced with many barriers to communicating effectively with physicians. Physicians may not accept recommendations and may, in fact, seem ungrateful to some of your interventions. Even when you do effect a change in physician behavior, you may not receive feedback that your efforts have been successful. Perhaps the next prescription the physician writes will show a change, even though the initial response to you indicated that a change would not be made.

Unfortunately, you are not always going to get a "pat on the back" for consultations with physicians. It is important to keep in mind, therefore, that consulting with physicians if problems arise or asking questions if something seems to be a problem must be done in spite of what the physician's reaction might be. To fail to consult a physician because of anticipated resistance reduces your professional role to one of subservience—one where you are willing to abdicate your responsibilities as a health professional or fail to act in the patient's best interest because you feel uncomfortable carrying out these patient care functions. While pharmacists seem to fear that physicians will not respond positively to therapeutic recommendations, the research evidence suggests just the opposite. Studies conducted in a number of different pharmacy practice environments indicate that, when pharmacists make suggestions to physicians for important therapeutic changes in a patient's drug treatment, in the vast majority of cases, pharmacist recommendations are accepted and implemented by physicians (Klopfer and Einarson, 1990; Deady et al., 1991; Berardo et al., 1994; Cooper, 1997; Gums et al., 1999). In any case, assertive pharmacists are aware at all times that their professional duty is to the patient and are assertive (and persistent) in seeing that the interests of patients are served.

When patient safety is compromised, it is the professional responsibility of the pharmacist to persist in trying to prevent or resolve problems. Research has found that more than 60% of medication errors are caused by problems in interpersonal communication (Joint Commission on Accreditation of Healthcare Organizations, 2005). More than one-half of health care workers in one survey reported seeing colleagues cutting corners or making mistakes, yet less than 10% reported saying anything about what they observed (Maxfield et al., 2006). The 10% who did speak up were also more satisfied with and more committed to their jobs. The "culture of safety" being mandated for health care organizations emphasizes the importance of approaching each other in an assertive manner when we have concerns about patient care processes taking place (Baker et al., 2005).

The World Health Organization Collaborating Centre for Patient Safety Solutions (2008) provides an online resource of safe practices for health care professionals to use to improve patient care. The "culture of silence" in the face of medical error that has historically governed collegial relationships is no longer tolerated in health care organizations.

Assertiveness and Employees

Please consider the following situation in Case Study 6.2. The manager of a hospital outpatient pharmacy has observed lately that one of the pharmacists has been creating problems. The manager's major concern is that the pharmacist is sometimes rude and abrupt with patients. Today, the manager overheard the pharmacist respond with obvious annoyance to a patient who expressed confusion about how to take her medication. The manager decides to talk privately with the pharmacist and provide feedback about his behavior.

CASE STUDY 6.2

Manager: I overheard your conversation with Mrs. Raymond this afternoon when you became impatient with her for not understanding instructions. I was upset because I didn't think you treated her with respect. I want you to treat patients with courtesy and not get so impatient and judgmental with them.

Pharmacist: Well, she had been complaining about how slow we were and then wouldn't pay attention when I was explaining the directions. I just got fed up.

Manager: I know that patients can be irritating, but I want you to treat them with respect.

Pharmacist: Well, we were so busy then that I just didn't have time to fool around.

Manager: I know it was hectic and you were feeling rushed today, but even then I want you to be more courteous.

Pharmacist: Well, it would certainly be easier to take time to be nice if you'd get enough pharmacists in here to cover the workload. Furthermore, if you'd train the techs better, they could be a lot more help to us.

Manager: Those things may be true, but right now I want to resolve the problem in the way you communicate with patients when you are irritated or hurried. I want you to agree to treat patients with respect, regardless of how busy we get. Will you do that?

Pharmacist: That's easier said than done.

Manager: Will you do it?

Pharmacy managers are responsible not only for how they communicate with patients, but also how other pharmacists and support personnel treat patients. They must make clear to all employees what is expected in the way of patient care. In the previous scene, the pharmacy manager used a number of assertive techniques in his conversation with the pharmacist. For one thing, he was specific about how he expected the pharmacist to behave and calmly repeated these expectations (called a "broken record" response) in spite of the pharmacist's excuses. He would not let himself be dragged off the point. He did not become defensive when the pharmacist attacked his performance as a manager. He might also have said, "I would like to discuss any ideas you might have about improving the training of techs another time, but right now I want to talk about the way you counsel patients." This would have let the pharmacist know that he was willing to listen to specific, constructive suggestions but not before the current problem was resolved.

The pharmacy manager also used appropriate feedback techniques. He told the pharmacist what he had observed about a specific behavior and what he wanted changed without attacking the pharmacist as a person. The manager did not label the pharmacist as being rude or thoughtless. Focusing feedback on what a person does is much less destructive than making personal judgments about him as a person. Such feedback also lets him know exactly what must be changed to improve his performance. The manager discussed the situation privately and soon after the incident occurred. He made "I" statements to provide feedback and define expectations, including "I overheard your conversation," "I was upset," and "I want you to treat patients with courtesy." Because of these "I" statements, the communication was less damaging to the relationship than if the manager had labeled or judged the pharmacist as a person ("You are rude") or if he had overgeneralized based on what he observed ("You *always* fly off the handle when we get busy here"). Dealing with the problem immediately was also much more effective than waiting until the annual job performance evaluations or until the problem had become so serious that more drastic action was required.

Many of the same guidelines that are useful in giving negative feedback apply as well to praise. A personal statement, such as telling a clerk, "I really appreciate your willingness to stay late tonight to help out" is more meaningful than a general statement (e.g., "You're a good clerk"). In addition, if positive feedback is an ongoing part of the relationship rather than something that only gets written on job performance evaluation forms, it is more effective. Too often, employees feel that the only time they get any feedback from their bosses is when they have done something wrong, which makes it much harder to accept the negative comments. Finally, your willingness to accept even negative feedback from employees (if it is constructive) can create an atmosphere of mutual respect. In the example above, the pharmacy manager conveyed both an assertive and empathic message when he said, "I know it was hectic and you were feeling rushed today, but even then I want you to be more courteous." He let the pharmacist know that he understood the feelings of frustration and at the same time insisted that certain standards be met in patient care.

Assertiveness and Employers

It is necessary to be assertive not only with your employees, but with your supervisors as well. We often "do as we are told" rather than identifying our goals in communication with supervisors and being persistent in pursuing those goals. As health professionals, we sometimes work in situations where supervisors share neither our professional identities nor the ethical standards we hold for patient care. It is necessary for us, then, to define what the professional standards for pharmacists are and to be assertive in insisting that we must meet those standards whatever our practice environment. In addition, we may be faced with a situation where we receive a negative evaluation or criticism of our performance by a supervisor. None of us enjoys hearing that someone is angry or disappointed with us for what we have done. Yet the criticisms we receive (and what we do in response to them) can lead to improved relationships with others, if we can avoid common pitfalls in our responses to criticism.

For some of us, our first response to criticism is to counterattack. The attitude is, "So what if I did make a mistake—I've seen you blow it a few times yourself." It is as if we can somehow "even the score" by criticizing the accuser. However, such responses mean we never have to deal with the possibly valid concerns others have about our behavior—we can always change the subject to their problems. In contrast to these aggressive responses, for more passive individuals, the initial response to criticism is to apologize excessively, give excuses, and generally act as if it is a catastrophe if someone is upset with us. Neither a passive nor aggressive response fosters problem solving.

When you are criticized, it is important to distinguish between (a) the truths people tell you about your behavior and (b) the judgments (the "wrong" or "bad" indictments) that they attach to your behavior. Often their judgments are arbitrary and are based on values you may not share. Even when you agree with the judgments made by someone criticizing you and think you were wrong, you must separate the foolish or careless thing you did from yourself as a person. The following are five responses that are helpful in various types of situations where criticism is levied.

GETTING USEFUL FEEDBACK

If the criticism is vague, it is necessary first to find out exactly what happened that led to the criticism. Uncovering the problem will provide you with specific feedback that may be useful to you in improving your performance. Therefore, before reacting to any problem that may be present, first be certain that you understand the exact nature of the problem. If a patient says that people in your pharmacy don't care about customers, find out exactly what happened that was upsetting and led to this conclusion. In order to know how to improve your service, you must have specific feedback that points out what changes might be needed.

AGREEING WITH CRITICISM

If you consider the criticism you receive to be valid, the most straightforward response is to acknowledge the mistake. If it is possible to counteract any of the damage, then that is done. In any case, avoid "Yes, but?" responses that try to excuse behavior but lead to increased annoyance on the part of the other person. "Yes, I am late for work a lot, but the traffic is so bad" usually leads to an escalation of the conflict ("You'll just have to leave home earlier!"). If you made a mistake or were wrong, acknowledge that. When you acknowledge mistakes and apologize for them, people have difficulty maintaining their anger. However, if you continue to make the same mistakes, the apologies will seem insincere and manipulative since you have not taken steps to prevent the problem from reoccurring. When you have issued a sincere apology, it also helps to report on efforts or changes you will make, so the problem is not repeated.

DISAGREEING WITH CRITICISM

Often criticism is not justified or is not appropriate because it is too broad; it is a personal attack rather than a criticism of specific behavior, or it is based on value judgments that you do not agree with. If you consider criticism unfair or unreasonable, it is important to state your disagreement and tell why. For example, you came in late to work this morning and your boss is fuming. During his attack, he says, "You're always late. Nobody around here cares about the patients waiting to get prescriptions filled."

It is important to say to him: "You're right, I was late this morning, and for that I apologize. But it is not true that I am always late. I know I was late one day last month but that is the only other time I can recall being late in the 2 years I have worked here. And it is not true that I do not care about our patients. I think the way I practice shows them my concern." Not speaking against something you consider to be a personal injustice or untruth leads to feelings of resentment and a loss of self-esteem for having kept quiet.

FOGGING

Fogging involves acknowledging the truth or possible truths in what people tell you about yourself while ignoring completely any judgments they might have implied by what they said. Manuel Smith (1975) outlined fogging as a basic assertive response to criticism. Let us see how this might apply in a pharmacy situation such as Case Study 6.3.

Such a response allows you to look at truths about your behavior *without* accepting the implied criticisms. The response makes it clear that your own standards guide your behavior without provoking a confrontation with the person levying the criticism. A fogging response differs from agreeing with the criticism. Agreeing with criticism includes acknowledging that you were wrong or behaved irresponsibly; you admit that your behavior failed to meet your own goals for yourself.

CASE STUDY 6.3

Supervisor: You spent a lot of time talking with that patient about a simple OTC choice.

Pharmacist: You're right. I did.

Supervisor: The other pharmacists let clerks do a lot of that sort of stuff.

Pharmacist: You're probably right. They may not spend as much time as I do on OTC consultations.

DELAYING A RESPONSE

If the criticism takes you by surprise and you are confused about how to respond, give yourself time to think about the problem before responding. Few conflict situations call for an immediate response. If you are too surprised or upset to think clearly about what you want to say, delay a response. Tell the person: "I want time to think about what you've told me, and then I'd like to sit down with you and try to clear up this problem. Could we discuss the situation this afternoon at the end of my shift?"

Assertiveness and Colleagues

The techniques for assertiveness with employers can also help you be more assertive with your colleagues. For example, the president of your local pharmacy association calls and asks you to serve as chairman of a new committee. You are interested in the committee but are not sure you have the time to chair it. Which of the following responses would you choose?

a. "Well, I'd really like to. I don't know. I guess I could if it doesn't take too much time."
b. "Why don't you ask Jim? He'd be good. If you can't find anyone else, maybe I could do it."
c. "I've given enough time to this organization. Everyone always comes to me. Let someone else do some work for a change."
d. "I'm interested in the committee, but I'm not sure I have time. Let me think about it tonight and I'll call you in the morning with my decision."

Response [d] seems most honest and assertive. We typically feel that we must respond immediately to situations that arise. Often the best response is to delay a response. It gives you time to decide what it is you really want to do. When you are facing a decision or when you are embroiled in a conflict, it is often best to say, "I want time to think. I'll get back to you." It is, of course, essential that you do get back to that person when you say you will and resolve the issue. Response [a] is a wishy-washy "yes." The problem with such a response is that you may say "yes" but never take responsibility for your decision. You

CASE STUDY 6.4

Association President: You would be perfect for the job. It is extremely important and I must have someone who knows the issues and stays on top of things.

Pharmacist: I appreciate that, but I won't be able to chair the committee this year.

President: I'll help with the workload. It shouldn't take more than an hour or so a week.

Pharmacist: That may be true, but I'm not willing to chair the committee right now.

President: Why not? Perhaps there is something we can do to resolve the problems you seem to think will come up in chairing the committee.

Pharmacist: The decision is really a personal one. I won't be able to chair the committee at this time.

may, instead, blame others for asking too much of you. The "yes" response, in this situation, was given because you found it difficult to say "no." Response [b] suggests that, if no one else will do it, you will feel that you must do it. You feel responsible for solving the president's problem by identifying someone to chair the committee. If he cannot find someone else, you will then feel obligated. The aggressive response, [c], is often the point a person comes to after a history of passive responses to similar requests. It sounds as if this person has said "yes" frequently in the past, felt overcommitted, and began to blame others for "asking" rather than taking personal responsibility for having said "yes." Others will make requests of you. It is up to you to say "yes" or "no" or to set limits on the extent of your involvement.

Let's now imagine a situation as in Case Study 6.4, where the president tries to coax or manipulate you into changing your "no" response to a "yes" response to his request to chair the committee. In this instance, the pharmacist again used a "broken record" response. He calmly repeated his "no" response without elaboration and with no rancor at the president's efforts to coax him into changing his mind. If the pharmacist had chosen to do so, he might have given an explanation for his decision, but he is not "obligated" to do so. The danger for passive people in giving an explanation is they seem to believe the president must agree that the decision is "justified" before they feel they have the right to say "no."

Summary

Assertiveness is a style of response that focuses on resolving conflicts in relationships in an atmosphere of mutual respect. To be assertive, each person must be able to directly and honestly convey "This is what I think," "This is how I feel about the situation," "This is what I want to have happen," or "This is what I am willing to do." This type of communication allows people to stand up for their own rights or for what they believe in without infringing on the rights of others. You also attempt to understand the other person's point of view even when there is disagreement. The focus is on problem solving rather than turning the conflict into a "win/lose" situation that damages the relationship.

You as a pharmacist are faced with numerous changes in your role within the health care system. If you are to lead these changes, to have a hand in shaping your own future, then you must be assertive in your communication with the other people you relate to in your professional practice.

REVIEW QUESTIONS

1. **Compare assertiveness to passivity and aggressiveness.**
2. **In what way(s) should pharmacists be assertive with patients? With physicians? With colleagues?**
3. **Describe a way to handle criticism without losing self-esteem or mutual respect.**
4. **How can assertiveness be used to resolve conflict?**
5. **What is "fogging"?**

REVIEW CASES

REVIEW CASE STUDY 6.1

A patient who is obviously in a hurry brings in a prescription to be filled. You are extremely busy and there is a 30-minute wait. When she is told this, she explodes, "That is ridiculous. It can't take that long to pour pills from a big bottle into a little bottle." When you start to explain about patient counseling, she says, "I've never had anyone talk with me about the prescriptions I get here. All you do is ask me to sign a form."

1. What special assertiveness skills might you use?
2. What is your role in this situation?

REFERENCES

Baker DP, Gustafson S, Beaubien J, et al. *Medical Teamwork and Patient Safety: The Evidence-based Relation*. 2005. Retrieved July 3, 2011 from http://www.ahrq.gov/qual/medteam.

Berardo DH, Kimberlin CL, McKenzie LC, Pendergast JF. Community pharmacists' documentation of intervention on drug-related problems of elderly patients. *Journal of Social and Administrative Pharmacy* 11:182–193, 1994.

Cooper J. Consultant pharmacist assessment and reduction of fall risk in nursing facilities. *Consultant Pharmacist* 12:1294–1298, 1303–1304, 1997.

Deady JE, Lepinski PW, Abramowitz PW. Measuring the ability of clinical pharmacists to effect drug therapy changes in a family practice clinic using prognostic indicators. *Hospital Pharmacy* 26: 93–97, 1991.

Gandhi TK, Weingart SN, Borus J, et al. Adverse drug events in ambulatory care. *New England Journal of Medicine* 348:1556–64, 2003.

Gums JG, Yancey RW, Hamilton CA, et al. Randomized, prospective study measuring outcomes after antibiotic therapy intervention by a multidisciplinary consult team. *Pharmacotherapy* 19: 1369–1377, 1999.

Joint Commission on Accreditation of Healthcare Organizations. The Joint Commission guide to improving staff communication. Oakbrook Terrace, IL: Joint Commission Resources; 2005.

Kaplan SH, Greenfield S, Ware JE Jr. Assessing the effects of physician-patient interactions on the outcomes of chronic disease. *Medical Care* 27:5110–5127, 1989.

Kaufman S, Elliott M, Shmueli D. Frames, framing and reframing. *The Conflict Resolution Information Source*. September 2003. Retrieved July 3, 2011 from http://crinfo.beyondintractability.org/essay/framing.

Kimberlin CL, Assa M, Rubin D, Zaenger P. Questions elderly patients have about on-going therapy: A pilot study to assist in communication with physicians. *Pharmacy World and Science* 23: 237–241, 2001.

Klopfer JD, Einarson TR. Acceptance of pharmacists' suggestions by prescribers: Literature review. *Hospital Pharmacy* 25:830–832,834–836, 1990.

Maxfield D, Grenny J, McMillan R, et al. *Silence Kills: The Seven Crucial Conversations for Healthcare*. Sponsored by the American Association of Critical-Care Nurses and VitalSmarts. Retrieved July 3, 2011 from http://psnet.ahrq.gov/resource.aspx?resourceID=1149.

Roter D. Patient participation in patient-provider interactions: The effects of patient question-asking on the quality of interactions, satisfaction and compliance. *Health Education Monographs* 5: 281–315, 1977.

Roter DL. Patient question asking in physician-patient interaction. *Health Psychology* 3:395–409, 1984.

Smith M. *When I Say No, I Feel Guilty*. New York, NY: Dial Press, 1975.

The World Health Organization Collaborating Centre for Patient Safety Solutions, 2008. Retrieved July 3, 2011 at http://www.ccforpatientsafety.org/Patient-Safety-Solutions.

Weingart SN, Pagovich O, Sands DZ, et al. What can hospitalized patients tell us about adverse events? Learning from patient-reported incidents. *Journal of General Internal Medicine* 20:830–836, 2005.

CHAPTER

7

Interviewing and Assessment

Overview

Patient assessment is an important aspect of patient care. Determining what patients understand about their medications, how they are taking their medications, how well their medications are working, and problems they perceive with their therapy are key elements to ensuring positive health outcomes. Gaining insight into patient understanding and actions assists pharmacists in planning an appropriate strategy for increasing understanding and appropriate use of medications. Interviewing is one of the most common methods used in patient assessment. Although interviewing is a common occurrence in pharmacy practice, the quality of the patient interview is an area that receives little attention by pharmacists. This chapter focuses on ways of improving patient assessment and the interviewing process. It addresses aspects of both informal questioning and the more formal, structured interview. Communication skills discussed include questioning, listening, using silence appropriately, and developing rapport.

Introduction

Pharmacists often must obtain information from patients as part of the patient assessment process. Inquiries range from simple requests, such as asking whether a patient is allergic to penicillin, to complex problems, such as determining whether a patient is taking a medication properly. Interviewing is an important component in the disease management process as pharmacists obtain information for therapeutic decision making. Effective interviewing also allows pharmacists to evaluate patient adherence to medication regimens by asking appropriate questions. At first glance, this process appears to be rather simple; it is something pharmacists do many times each day. However, research and experience have shown that interviewing is a complex process in need of more attention, because the quality of the information received is not always optimal.

The accuracy, depth, and breadth of information provided by a patient in an interview are influenced by many factors, such as the patient's perception of the interview and the physical environment in which the interview takes place—factors that have been discussed earlier. However, the accuracy of the patient assessment is also influenced by the interviewing process and by the way you ask patients questions.

One of the first steps in the patient assessment process should be to determine not only what medications patients may take, but also what patients already know about their medications and health-related problems. Determining how much patients know is necessary because patient education strategies vary depending on the depth of understanding patients already possess. Patients who are very familiar with their medications have different needs than those who know relatively little. You become more efficient if you can identify those individuals who need extra counseling. It is inefficient to repeat information that patients already understand. By using an initial assessment technique, you essentially use the patient as a database to determine what information is already mastered. You then "fill in the void" with the information you think is important for a particular patient.

The process of interviewing goes beyond asking a series of preplanned questions in a certain order. Although this approach may be effective in some aspects of pharmacy care, such as screening for hypertension, it may not be the most appropriate approach in other situations, such as when patients are reluctant to talk about their problems (Bernstein and Bernstein, 1980). The basic skills discussed in this unit can be used in a variety of settings or situations and, if used properly, can greatly enhance the efficiency of the interview and the quality of information obtained.

Components of an Effective Interview

As mentioned earlier, conducting an effective interview is not a simple process. The interviewing process contains several critical components that should be mastered. The process is somewhat analogous to learning to drive a car. At first, you must learn specific skills, such as applying the brakes properly or using the rearview mirror. Once these skills have been learned, the process becomes automatic and rather simple—until you have an accident. Then you must analyze what went wrong with your skills (e.g., you didn't use the turn signal, or you miscalculated your speed on a curve); the driving skill is then corrected or relearned, and you continue on safely. The same is true with effective interviewing. Certain communication and interviewing skills need to be mastered and used, or you are likely to have an incomplete or otherwise unproductive interview. The problems in the interviewing process can be minor (e.g., you miss one piece of information) or major (e.g., you fail to identify an important adverse effect the patient is experiencing from a medication). By considering the elements of effective interviewing in this chapter, you will be able to avoid problems and analyze what went wrong if a problem does arise.

LISTENING

In general, people are better senders of information than receivers of information. We have been taught how to improve our verbal and written communication skills, but not our listening skills. Thus, we must concentrate much harder on the listening component of the communication process. Nothing will end an interview faster than having patients realize that you are not listening to them. Listening skills were discussed in depth in Chapter 5. In addition, see Box 7.1 for other suggestions for how to improve your listening skills.

BOX 7.1 Listening Techniques for the Interview Process

- **Stop talking.** You can't listen while you are talking.
- **Get rid of distractions.** These break your concentration.
- **Use good eye contact** (i.e., look at the other person). This helps you concentrate and shows the other person that you are indeed listening.
- **React to ideas, not to the person.** Focus on what is being said and not on whether you like the person.
- **Read nonverbal messages.** These may communicate the same or a different message than the one given verbally.
- **Listen to how something is said.** The tone of voice and rate of speech also transmit part of the message.
- **Provide feedback (briefly summarize your understanding) to clarify any messages.** This also shows that you are listening and trying to understand.

PROBING

Another important communication skill is learning to ask questions in a way that elicits the most accurate information. This technique is called "probing." Probing is the use of questions to elicit needed information from patients or to help clarify their problems or concerns. Asking questions seems to be a straightforward task, which it is in most situations. However, several things should be considered before asking a question. The phrasing of the question is important. Patients are often put on the defensive by questions. For instance, "why" type questions can make people feel that they have to justify their reason for doing a certain thing. It is usually better to use "what" or "how" type of questions. For example, people might become defensive if asked "Why do you miss doses of medication?" instead of "What causes you to miss doses of medication?"

In addition, the timing of the question is important. Several questions in succession may leave the patient with a sense of being interrogated and, therefore, may raise the level of defensiveness. The patient should be allowed to finish answering the current question before proceeding to the next one. In addition, leading questions should be avoided. These questions strongly imply an expected answer (e.g., "You don't usually forget to take the medication, do you?" or "You take this three times a day with meals, right?"). These questions lead patients into saying what they think you want to hear rather than what the truth may be.

To conduct an effective interview, it is important to understand the differences between closed-ended and open-ended questions. A closed-ended question can be answered with either a "yes" or "no" response or with a few words at most. On the other hand, an open-ended question neither limits the patient's response nor induces defensiveness. For example, a closed-ended question would be "Has your doctor told you how to take this medication?" The patient may only respond with a "yes" and not provide any useful information to you. On the other hand, an open-ended question would be "How has your doctor told you to take this medication?" The phrasing of this question allows patients to state exactly how they perceive that the medication should be taken. Proper open-ended questions are harder to formulate than closed-ended questions, but they are more crucial in obtaining complete information and in decreasing the patient's defensiveness by conveying a willingness on your part to listen. With an open-ended question, you are allowing patients to present information in their own words.

Closed-ended questions reduce the patient's degree of openness and cause the patient to become more passive during the interviewing process because you are doing most of the talking. Closed-ended questions also enable patients to avoid specific subjects and emotional expression. Such questions can connote an air of interrogation and impersonality. For this reason, closed-ended questions are referred to as "pharmacist-centered questions." Open-ended questions do not require the other person to respond in your frame of reference. Open-ended questions permit open expression and for this reason are sometimes referred to as "patient-centered questions." Closed-ended questions are necessary and are indeed useful; however, open-ended questions are less likely to result in misunderstanding, and they tend to promote rapport.

You may find a combination of open-ended and closed-ended questions most efficient in your practice. Patient encounters may be initiated with an open-ended question, followed by more directed, closed-ended questions. For example, if you want to know whether Mr. Raymond is experiencing bothersome side effects from his antihypertensive medication, you may say, "How have you been feeling since starting this medicine?" or "What things have you noticed since beginning this medication?" If symptoms that may indicate a side effect are mentioned, follow-up questions are used to assess the severity of the adverse effects, such as "How bothersome are these side effects?" If necessary, open-ended questioning can be followed by more direct questions that focus on specific side effects often associated with a particular medication, such as "Do you have trouble sleeping?," "Do you feel weak?," "Do you feel tired?," and so on.

Experience has found that open-ended questions are more effective in assessing patient understanding. The Indian Health Service has developed an effective patient education program that uses a series of open-ended questions during the patient assessment process (Gardner et al., 1991). For new prescriptions, the questions "What did your doctor tell you the medication is for?," "How did your doctor tell you to take the medication?," and "What did your doctor tell you to expect?" are suggested as a way to structure the assessment of patient understanding of new prescriptions (Gardner et al., 1991). Open-ended questions provide an opportunity for you to assess whether or not the patient understands the key elements of drug therapy (see Box 7.2).

Based on these assessments of patient knowledge, you will be able to develop a strategy to deal with patients' lack of knowledge or misconceptions about drug use. You may provide additional information, calm their fears, and provide necessary encouragement. You may also give them take-home written material and follow up with a phone call.

Whatever the purpose of the patient interview, be aware of when and how you ask a question. The ultimate test is this: Will the question I am about to ask be

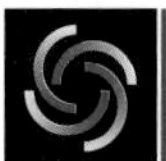

BOX 7.2 Key Elements of Drug Therapy

- Purpose of medication
- How the medication works
- Dose/interval
- Duration of therapy
- Goals of therapy
- How effectiveness will be monitored
- Adverse effects and strategies to deal with these events
- Drug-specific issues

helpful in understanding the other person's drug therapy needs and problems? Open-ended questions elicit more complete and unabridged information that does not squeeze the patient into your perspective. Open-ended questions convey a willingness to listen. Conversely, closed-ended questions reduce openness, can encourage passivity, and can lead to patient avoidance of emotional expression. Open-ended questions are almost always better than closed-ended questions because they yield more information. Of course, in some situations a simple "yes" or "no" answer will be necessary. Closed-ended questions help you collect specific clinical data efficiently. It takes practice to develop a good questioning technique that uses a combination of both closed- and open-ended questions to move the interview to its conclusion. Tact must also be developed when you use open-ended questions to prevent patients from wandering off into subject areas that might not be relevant to the situation.

ASKING SENSITIVE QUESTIONS

Some questions you ask patients may be particularly sensitive. Questions assessing adherence, alcohol use, or use of recreational drugs may be difficult to ask. Assessment of effects (including side effects) of medications that relate to sexual functioning or sexually transmitted diseases may also require a diplomatic approach. There are a number of techniques that can make such questions easier to ask.

Before asking a question about a sensitive topic, let the patient know that the behaviors or problems you are asking about are common. If you acknowledge that many of your patients have similar problems, it makes the issue seem less threatening. For example, say to a patient "It is very difficult to take a medication consistently, day after day. Nearly everyone will miss a dose of medication once in a while" before asking specific questions about adherence. Framing the question in this way can make it feel safe for patients to admit they are having difficulty adhering to a medication regimen. Patients do not fear that you will judge them harshly for missing doses of medication if you preface your question with an accepting statement. Gardner et al. (1995) refer to these remarks as "universal statements." Examples of universal statements they identify include "This is a very common concern...," "Frequently my patients have difficulty...," and "Everybody has trouble with..."

Another technique for reducing the threat of sensitive questions is to ask whether the situation has ever, at any time, occurred and then ask about the current situation. For example, if you decide that you must assess use of illicit drugs, you may phrase the question in the following way: "Other types of drugs, such as marijuana, are commonly used. People might use it to relax or with friends at a party. Have you at any time in your life smoked marijuana?" If the answer is "yes," the follow-up question might be "To put things in a more recent time frame, have you smoked marijuana during the past year?" Questions about frequency of use and use of other drugs could follow. A similar process could be used to obtain precise information on adherence with a prescribed regimen, such as use of antiretroviral agents where strict adherence is important. Asking first whether the patient has ever missed a dose of a medication and then progressing to estimates of the number of doses missed in the last week may make the information the patient provides more reliable.

In addressing these issues, use of simple, clear-cut questions and a matter-of-fact manner are critical. The way you phrase the question and your tone of voice should be no different for a question on alcohol consumption than for a question on use of an over-the-counter (OTC) product.

In structuring the interview, it helps to embed more threatening topics among less threatening topics and to ask more "personal" questions later in the interview. For example, questions about alcohol consumption may be better accepted by the patient if they follow questions about caffeine consumption.

If patients seem reluctant to address an issue, it helps to discuss the reason why you are asking a particular question. You might use a statement such as: "People often do not think of alcohol as a drug, but there are many medications that can interact with alcohol. I ask about alcohol use so that I can help you prevent problems with the medications you take." If patients understand the reason for a question, they are more likely to respond honestly. If they do not know the reason, they may make assumptions about why questions are being asked. Unfortunately, the assumptions they make may be more damaging than the truth. In any case, before asking *any* question, and especially one that may be sensitive, be sure that the question is necessary and that you have a clear need for the information in your efforts to help the patient.

USE OF SILENCE

Another skill that you must learn in order to be an effective interviewer is the art of using silence appropriately. During the interview, there will be times when neither you nor the patient will speak, especially in the early moments. You must learn to treat these pauses as necessary parts of the process and not be uncomfortable with them. Many times, the patient needs time to think about or react to the information you have provided or the question you have asked. Interrupting the silence destroys the opportunity for the patient to think about this material. On the other hand, the pause might be due to the fact that the patient did not understand the question completely. In this situation, the question should be restated or rephrased. At the same time, too much silence when a patient is expressing feelings such as fear or depression may be interpreted by the patient as rejection. In this case, the patient may be seeking an indication that you understand the concerns expressed. Responding with empathy is a necessary component of any communication you have with a patient.

In any event, you should avoid the temptation to fill empty spaces in the interview with unnecessary talk. In fact, some studies have found that the more the "talk ratio" is in favor of the person being interviewed (i.e., the patient does more of the talking), the more likely it is that the interview will be successful. Thus, the patient should be able to relax and be allowed time to think during the necessary pauses in the interview process.

BOX 7.3 Interview Considerations

- Type of information
- Type of environment
- Starting the interview
- Ending the interview

ESTABLISHING RAPPORT

Successful interviews are marked by a high degree of rapport between the two parties. Rapport is built mainly on mutual consideration and respect. You can aid this process by using good eye contact, by using a sincere, friendly greeting, by being courteous during the discussion, and by not stereotyping or prejudging the patient. Each patient must be seen as a unique individual. As mentioned earlier, patients' perceptions of you will influence their relationship with you. Thus, it is critical that you initiate the interaction in a friendly, professional manner.

Interviewing as a Process

Proper planning and sequencing of the interview are essential in carrying out an effective patient assessment. Before an interview is started, several decisions must be made regarding how it will be structured. The type of approach usually depends on the type of information desired and the environment and time available for it. See Box 7.3.

TYPE OF INFORMATION

Before the interview begins, you should determine the amount and type of information desired. In other words, what exactly do you want to accomplish? For example, if you need to find out specific pieces of information, you will want to have more control over the interview process. This is referred to as the *directed* interview approach. However, if the outcome is unknown or somewhat ambiguous, you need to use a more *nondirective* approach. This approach allows the interview to become more free-flowing; the points of discussion are raised by the patient rather than by you. When you use this approach, you hope the problem or concern will surface, allowing you to deal with it. In the nondirective approach, open-ended questions should be used more frequently than closed-ended questions. However, even in the directed approach you can ask an initial open-ended question to assess patient understanding as discussed earlier.

TYPE OF ENVIRONMENT

Planning for the interview must include consideration of the type of environment available. The environment is critical, because one of the fundamental principles of interviewing is to provide as much privacy as possible. Research has shown that the degree of privacy is related to many critical outcomes of the interview process (e.g., the level of patient understanding of the information provided and the degree of adherence with the treatment regimen). As the privacy of the setting increases, the amount of information retained by the patient increases, along with the likelihood that the patient will take the prescribed medication appropriately (Beardsley et al., 1977). Privacy also allows both you and the patient to express personal concerns, to ask difficult questions, to listen more effectively, and to share honest opinions. Unfortunately, the setting of the interview in many pharmacies—over a busy prescription counter or in other areas where distractions abound—is not always optimal. Before you begin the interview, interruptions should be reduced as much as possible. A partition at the end of the prescription counter, a special room, or a consulting area can provide the necessary privacy.

STARTING THE INTERVIEW

After considering the type of environment available and the type of information desired, you should start the interview by greeting patients by name and introducing yourself to patients if you do not know them. This helps establish rapport with the patient. You should also state the purpose of the interview, outline what will happen during the interview, and put the patient at ease. The purpose of the interview should be stated in terms of the benefit to the patient. The amount of time needed, the subjects to be covered, and the final outcome should be mentioned so the patient has a clear understanding of the process. For example, a pharmacist seeing a patient for the first time might say:

Hello, Mr. Pearson, I'm Jane Bradley, the pharmacist (the introduction). Since you are new to our pharmacy, I would like to ask you a few quick questions about the medications you are now taking (the subjects to be covered). This will take about 5 to 10 minutes (the amount of time needed) and will allow me to create a drug profile so that I can keep track of all the medications you are taking. This will help us identify potential problems with new medications that might be prescribed for you (the purpose/outcome).

Such a beginning allows you to define the limits and expectations of the interview. After the interview is started, the following suggestions will help you conduct a more efficient interview:

1. Avoid making recommendations during the information-gathering phases of the interview. Such recommendations prevent the patient from giving you all the needed information and can interfere with your ability to grasp the "big picture" of patient need.

2. Similarly, do not jump to conclusions or rapid solutions without hearing all the facts.
3. Do not shift from one subject to another until each subject has been followed through.
4. Guide the interview using a combination of open- and closed-ended questions.
5. Similarly, keep your goals clearly in mind, but do not let them dominate how you go about the interview. Flexibility is required so that you can reinforce patients for bringing up issues they consider important. In order for the communication to be patient centered, the patient must have some control over the communication process itself.
6. Determine the patient's ability to learn specific information in order to guide you in your presentation of the material. Reading ability, language proficiency, and vision or hearing impairments would all influence the techniques you use in interviewing and counseling a patient.
7. Maintain objectivity by not allowing the patient's attitudes, beliefs, or prejudices to influence your thinking.
8. Use good communication skills, especially the probing, listening, and feedback components.
9. Be aware of the patient's nonverbal messages, because these signal how the interview is progressing.
10. Depending upon your relationship with the patient, move from general to more specific questions and less personal to more personal subjects. This may remove some of the patient's initial defensiveness.
11. Note taking should be as brief as possible.

ENDING THE INTERVIEW

Bringing the interview to a close is often more difficult than starting the interview. It is a crucial part of the interview process because a person's evaluation of the entire interview and your performance may be based on the final statements. People seem to remember best what was said last. Therefore, care should be taken not to end the interview abruptly or to rush the patient out the door.

If you have provided important information to the patient, you should determine whether or not the patient understood the material correctly at the end of the interaction. For example, you could say to the patient: "I want to make sure I have explained everything clearly. Please summarize for me the most important things to remember about this new medicine." Other simple open-ended questions, such as "When you get home, how are you going to take this medication?" or "What side effects are you going to look for when taking this medication?" will allow patients to reflect on what they heard and understood. Gardner et al. (1991) refer to this part of the interview as the "Final Verification" of patient understanding.

To conclude the interview, you will want to briefly summarize the key information provided by the patient. A summary allows both parties the opportunity to review exactly what has been discussed and helps clarify any misunderstanding.

It is essential that both people agree about what has been said. A summary sets the stage for future patient contact and expectations that you both have of one another. A summary also tactfully hints to the patient that the interview is ending. In conjunction with a summary, you can use nonverbal cues to indicate to the patient that the interview is over. For instance, you could get up from the chair or change your stance in such a way that indicates that you need to move on. A simple closed-ended question such as: "Do you have any further questions?" or a statement such as "I've enjoyed talking with you. If you think of something you forgot to mention or have questions when you get home, please give me a call" may also be useful.

The ending of the interview is a good time for you to reassure the patient about a particular problem. However, this should not be false assurance, such as "Everything is going to turn out okay" or "Don't worry about it." Instead, you should state, "I will try to help things get better for you" along with specific action or follow-up you will implement. Tell the patient how and when you would like to contact him or her (e.g., by telephone call in 1 week) to make sure that a problem identified has been resolved and the patient is responding well to any therapeutic changes that have been made. With a new prescription, follow-up is also important to identify and resolve possible problems early in treatment. Waiting until a refill visit to find out how a patient is doing with a new prescription is often not the most timely or effective way to monitor response to a medication.

Before terminating the interview, you should reflect on whether the goals of the interview were accomplished and what should be done if they were not. After the patient has left, you should assess in your own mind what went well and what could have been done differently to help you continue to improve your interviewing skills. Finally, key information must be documented as part of the patient record. The information that should be documented from a patient interview is described later in this chapter.

Interviewing in Pharmacy Practice

Interviews in pharmacy practice are often thought of in terms of complete medication history interviews. However, if an interview is thought of as a process of obtaining information from patients to assess potential medication-related problems, there are a number of activities pharmacists engage in that can be thought of as interviewing. Assessing the health problems a patient presents before making an OTC recommendation is a targeted interview. Evaluating a patient's response to treatment and perceived problems related to medication therapy during a refill visit is another example of an interview. The specific questions that are asked may vary somewhat because the purpose of the interview varies, but the skills involved in gathering information from patients to assess problems and needs remain the same.

In assessing medication therapy, such as in a medication history interview, it is necessary to ensure you have a complete listing of medications being taken, including prescriptions, OTCs, herbals, and other complementary and alternative medicines. For each medication, an assessment is made of (a) the patient perception of the purpose of the medication, (b) the way the medication is actually being used by the patient, (c) patient-perceived effectiveness (along with specific information on indicators of effectiveness derived from physician reports to the patient or patient self-monitoring of response), and (d) problems the patient perceives with therapy.

It is also important to ask patients about health problems they have been experiencing or ones that have been diagnosed but that are not currently being treated with medication. You want to uncover health problems that should be brought to the attention of providers but, for whatever reasons, have not already been discussed. Perhaps the patient does not consider the problem "important" enough, or perhaps the costs associated with office visits and treatment are of concern. Fears related to an imagined diagnosis may prevent patients from seeking care.

In other cases, a patient may have received a diagnosis (e.g., type 2 diabetes) that is being treated by means other than medication (e.g., diet and exercise). Additionally, patients may have received a diagnosis and been prescribed a medication for a chronic condition that they decided on their own not to use or to discontinue taking. Medication-related problems include not only problems with medications being taken, but also drug therapy that is needed but is not being received by the patient.

Case study 7.1 is an example of an interview in a community pharmacy setting. A new patient, Robert Evans, comes to the pharmacy and presents a prescription for hydrochlorothiazide (HCTZ). The pharmacist, Ed Robinson, initiates a brief interview. In Case Study 7.1, the goal of the questions the pharmacist asked Mr. Evans was to establish a medication record along with a record of current medical conditions. In addition, the pharmacist sought to obtain the information needed to assess the effectiveness of and problems with the treatment of current conditions. The interview was limited, focusing on information needed to assess problems with current therapy and to uncover health problems that are not being treated with medications. For the medications the patient was currently taking, assessment focused on the following:

- Patient understanding of purpose
- Actual patterns of use and possible problems with use, including nonadherence
- Perceived effectiveness along with specific information from physician monitoring and patient self-monitoring that could provide additional "evidence" the pharmacist could use to assess patient response to treatment
- Patient perceptions of problems with therapy

Patient-perceived problems may include side effects experienced, cost concerns, inconvenience of dosing schedules, and so on. Phrasing a very open-ended question about problems allows patients to discuss anything they might perceive as problematic. More direct or closed-ended, follow-up questions about specific issues of concern, such as whether the patient has experienced symptoms that

CASE STUDY 7.1

Ed: Hello. Are you Robert Evans?

Robert: Yes.

Ed: Mr. Evans, I'm Ed Robinson, the pharmacist here. I would like to sit down with you and talk about the medications you currently take. This can help us identify problems you might be having with your drug therapy. We can talk while the technician is filling your prescription. Do you have about 10 minutes?

Robert: Sure. I was going to wait for my prescription anyway.

Ed: Let's start with the prescription you brought in today. What has your doctor told you about this medicine?

Robert: Dr. Carter told me I have high blood pressure. This isn't the first prescription for this HCTZ medicine though. I've been taking it about 3 years. My old prescription ran out of refills. Dr. Carter gave me a new one today.

Ed: When were you first diagnosed with high blood pressure?

Robert: About 3 years ago. I don't remember what my blood pressure was, but the doc said it was high.

Ed: Are you taking any other medications for your high blood pressure?

Robert: No, just the one.

Ed: How well has the HCTZ medication worked for you?

Robert: It has done the trick. Dr. Carter says I'm doing great.

Ed: That must be encouraging to hear! Tell me, what was your blood pressure today when you saw Dr. Carter?

Robert: 125/85. I take my blood pressure myself every day and it always stays around that.

Ed: It's a great idea to keep track of your own blood pressure. How often do you see Dr. Carter to have your blood pressure checked by him?

Robert: I see him every 6 months. At first it was every couple of months, but he said I am doing so well now, he doesn't have to see me as often.

Ed: That's great. Tell me, what problems have you had with this medication?

Robert: I haven't had any problems.

Ed: Have you noticed any side effects or symptoms you think are related to the medication?

Robert: I haven't had any side effects. I really haven't had any problems with the medication.

Ed: In terms of how you have been taking the HCTZ, describe your schedule on a typical day.

Case Study 7.1, cont.

Robert: I swallow it with my orange juice when I eat breakfast.

Ed: It's sometimes difficult to take a medication every day, day after day. How often would you say you miss a dose in a typical week?

Robert: I never miss. I fill up one of those weekly pill containers every Sunday and keep it beside the cereal in the cupboard so I remember to take it. Last time I forgot to take it was a month or so ago. I had gone to a restaurant for breakfast and I forgot it that morning. But that hardly ever happens.

Ed: Sounds like you really stay on top of it. Are there other things you do to help you control your high blood pressure?

Robert: Dr. Carter put me on a diet and exercise program. I've lost over 50 pounds in the past couple of years. I don't eat a lot of salt either.

Ed: You're really doing what you need to do to keep your blood pressure down. Do you have any questions or concerns about your medicine or your high blood pressure?

Robert: No. I think I've been doing fine. I've gotten used to taking a pill every day.

Ed: If any concerns do come up in the future, please let me know. Next, let me ask about other prescription medications you might currently be taking?

Robert: I don't take anything else. One drug is all I take.

Ed: I see. Let me switch to over-the-counter products that you can buy without a prescription.

Robert: I don't take anything. Maybe Tylenol once a year for a headache. Doc told me not to take anything for a cold without checking with him or a pharmacist. I don't like taking drugs, so I don't use that stuff you can buy in a grocery store.

Ed: Any vitamins or herbal products?

Robert: Nope.

Ed: Do you have any health concerns or other conditions a doctor has told you about that you are not treating with medication?

Robert: None. I'm healthy except for the high blood pressure.

Ed: That's good to hear. Do you have any allergies, especially reactions to medications?

Robert: No, no allergies at all.

At this point, the pharmacist might conclude the interview by thanking the patient for taking the time to answer questions, making sure there is not another issue related to drug therapy the patient might want to discuss. Finally, he can make himself available by telephone or in person if the patient wants to discuss drug therapy or any health concerns in the future.

may indicate adverse reactions to the medication, may be indicated to assure that such an important issue is not overlooked.

In Case Study 7.1, the pharmacist made the judgment to conduct a focused, brief interview. However, more extensive data gathering may be desirable or a series of interviews over time may be necessary to obtain a more complete picture of the patient's medical conditions and treatment needs. For example, a more intensive interviewing process has been described as a key component of the Pharmacist's Work-up of Drug Therapy (Cipolle et al., 1998). This workup is designed to thoroughly evaluate a patient's drug-related needs and drug therapy problems. Information is obtained in a number of areas, including demographics and family history, past medical history, current medical problems, allergies and adverse drug reactions, lifestyle issues related to health, immunization history, a medication record of current and recent past medication use, and a review of systems for thorough assessment of drug-related needs.

One benefit of conducting a lengthier, in-depth interview is that you will be better able to obtain information about a patient's quality of life (QOL), which is an important measure of therapeutic success. Patients' QOL beliefs may help you determine how they define therapeutic success. To you, the therapy may appear to be working while to your patient it is not, since it has not improved his or her ability to engage in desired activities. Using probing questions related to QOL

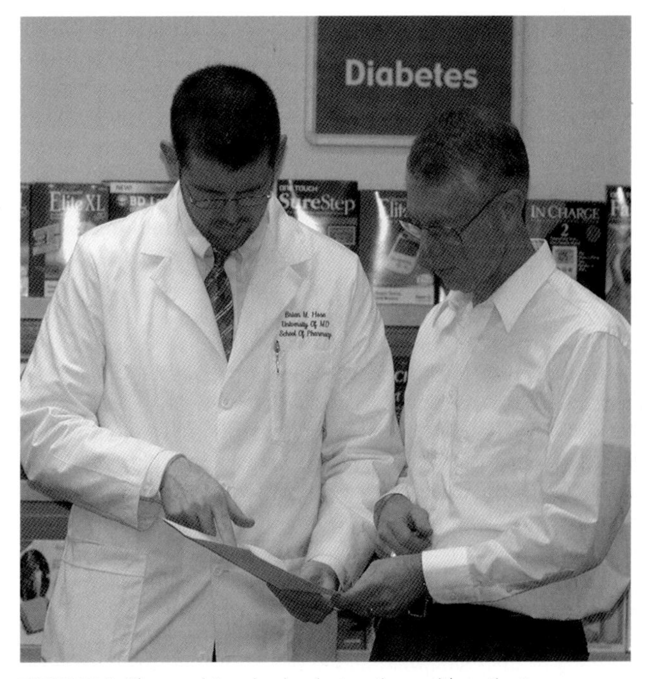

FIGURE 7-1. Pharmacist reviewing instructions with patient.

functioning during the interview process allows you to explore important factors related to QOL and satisfaction with therapy.

Interviewing and Patient-Reported Outcomes

When we hear the term "drug therapy monitoring" we may immediately think of clinical monitoring using lab values or monitoring devices. However, monitoring for many medications relies wholly or primarily on patient self-reports of therapeutic effect. Evaluation of depression, pain, anxiety, insomnia, migraine headaches, and menopausal symptoms are based on patient self-report of symptoms. Management of other diverse conditions, including asthma, seizure control, arthritis, COPD (chronic obstructive pulmonary disease), gastrointestinal disorders, and ADHD (attention deficit hyperactivity disorder), rely on patient or caregiver reports to diagnose the condition and monitor therapy effectiveness. Evaluation of tolerability or adverse effects of almost any drug therapy must include self-report or caregiver report of symptoms. In addition, use of self-monitoring devices and patient communication of results are crucial in monitoring a number of chronic diseases, including diabetes, hypertension, and increasingly, anticoagulation therapy.

The term "patient-reported outcome" in the literature is usually used to refer to quality-of-life outcomes or patient satisfaction with care. However, the term can be understood more broadly as any outcome reported subjectively by the patient or caregiver. In pharmacy practice, outcome assessment consists largely of patient reports of symptom experience, functional physical and mental status, and perceived changes in health status. In addition, having patients report on physician-conducted monitoring can help the pharmacist assess therapeutic response as well as patient understanding of therapy goals and the monitoring process. These patient reports also can provide information on the regularity with which lab values are obtained and therapeutic progress monitored by the physician. While some patients may not have specific information on lab values, others will be able to report INR (international normalized ratio), HbA1c (hemoglobin A1c test), viral load, or cholesterol values and have a sophisticated level of understanding of the management of their disease and therapy.

Research has examined which patient-reported outcomes are used as efficacy endpoints in product labeling for drugs newly approved by the U.S. Food and Drug Administration (Willke et al., 2004). The patient self-reported endpoint measures involved health-related QOL, health status, event logs, symptom reports, adherence reports, and satisfaction with treatment. Patient-reported outcomes were endpoints in 30% of product labels reviewed. Some therapies rely exclusively on patient-reported outcomes to measure both effectiveness and adverse effects.

Depression is one condition where both diagnosis and monitoring of effectiveness rely on patient self-report of symptoms. Often depressed persons initially self-treat depression-related symptoms such as pain, insomnia, and gastrointestinal distress. Pharmacists may, in such situations, be instrumental in conducting initial screening of such symptoms and referring the patient if depression seems probable. A quick screen for possible depression involves the following two yes/no questions: During the past month, have you often been bothered by:

1. Feeling down, depressed, or hopeless?
2. Having little interest or pleasure in doing things? (Whooley et al., 1997)

Persons who answer "yes" to either question should be referred for a more thorough assessment by a clinician. For patients beginning antidepressant therapy, it will be important to assess the symptoms they have been experiencing that they think are associated with the depression. The frequency, duration, and severity of symptoms identified, such as waking up every night for a month and not being able to get back to sleep, will help you identify the particular symptoms experienced by the individual patient initiating drug therapy. This information can then serve as the baseline by which to evaluate response to therapy as treatment progresses.

Pain is another condition that relies almost exclusively on self-report of symptoms. A familiar scale for measuring pain intensity is the Visual Analogue Scale (Wallerstein, 1984), which says to the patient "If 0 is 'no pain' and 10 is 'worst possible pain,' how would you rate your pain now?" and "What is the worst your pain has been in the last week?" In addition, assessment should establish patient goals for therapy with a question such as "What level of pain control on the 0 to 10 scale would you need to allow you to carry out the activities you desire?"

In addition to interviewing patients about therapeutic outcomes, resources have been developed to facilitate patient report of response to therapy. These resources include diaries and forms to document use of medications, effectiveness of therapy, and adverse effects or other problems experienced. The Write Track (1997) assists cancer patients in documenting response to medications being taken, including pain medications. In addition, the diary entries document side effects of chemotherapy and other medications being taken. This documentation is shared with providers in order to facilitate the joint decision-making process, including planning when to schedule chemotherapy. Use of this system of monitoring adverse events while undergoing chemotherapy was found, according to patients, to be valuable and one they would recommend to others with cancer.

For *any* therapy, monitoring involves knowing the key indicators of effectiveness for each particular therapy, the baseline values for the patient, and the goals of therapy for the patient. This information is required to determine effectiveness of treatment or progress toward treatment goals. The systematic gathering of information to evaluate therapy is necessary whether the measures involve lab values or patient self-reported response.

Documenting Interview Information

The documentation process is a means of assuring continuity of care to patients. The information documented in a note becomes the "institutional memory" of the care that has been provided. This will assist in your own follow-up care as well as communicate to colleagues about the care you have provided to a particular patient. Such communication is essential to the functioning of a health care team.

A format for documentation that is familiar to health care professionals is the SOAP note. SOAP is an acronym for Subjective, Objective, Assessment, and Plan. Subjective information is that information reported by the patient or patient caregiver, such as symptom experience or self-report of adherence. Objective information is that provided by a lab test or physical exam. If a pharmacist, as part of an interview with a hypertensive patient, takes the patient's blood pressure, for example, this would be documented as objective information. The Assessment section includes a description of any medication-related problem identified during the interview. For example, a problem may be lack of therapeutic response secondary to reported nonadherence. The assessment should be as specific as possible in order to lead logically to the plan to resolve the problem (the "P" portion of the SOAP note). For example, nonadherence caused by inability to pay for the prescription requires a different intervention plan from nonadherence caused by forgetting doses.

By the same token, if you obtained information indicating that the patient was responding well to treatment and had no problems with a medication regimen, this information should be noted and the assessment documented that no problems were identified. This serves to document that the assessment was made. Lack of information on a regimen could be interpreted by a third party to mean that you asked no questions about that regimen and an assessment was not made. To make sure communication with colleagues is unambiguous, document findings that indicate appropriate use, adequate response, and no problems with the regimen.

Once the assessment of a problem is made, based on the subjective and objective information included in the note, the plan should detail the actions to be taken to resolve the problem. The plan should include both an intervention plan and a monitoring plan. These plans must be specific. Specify action that will be taken by you, the date the action will be taken, and when follow-up with the patient will occur. For example, an intervention may require a consultation with a prescribing physician for a change in therapy. Document when the physician will be contacted, how (e.g., by phone), what will be recommended, and how the change in therapy will be initiated. The description of the initiation of a change should specify the new regimen as well as who will inform and educate the patient about the changes in therapy. In addition, the plan would document when follow-up with the patient will be initiated to assess the effects of any changes or recommendations made to improve therapy.

Interviewing Using the Telephone

Many times you need to collect information from patients by telephone. In light of the importance of the telephone, you should strive to maximize its effective use. Effective telephone skills can also help create a positive image for your pharmacy and lend support to your professional credibility. In addition, proficient telephone communication can contribute to personnel productivity and, ultimately, to the professional success of your pharmacy. The following should be considered during this type of interaction:

1. Cue yourself to smile before you pick up the telephone. Your friendly attitude will be transmitted through the tone, pitch, volume, and inflection of your voice.
2. If at all possible, answer the telephone or have a fellow employee answer it within the first three or four rings.
3. Identify the pharmacy and yourself, providing both your name and position (e.g., "Professional Pharmacy, Jane Jones speaking. May I help you?"). While it may appear burdensome to identify yourself fully to every caller, you should keep in mind that each call may represent the first contact the caller has with you and your pharmacy. Even if it is not the first contact, each call is a uniquely important communication for the caller and should be treated with respect.
4. Give your full attention to the call. Nothing is more irritating to callers than to be given the impression that they are competing for your attention.
5. Ask for the caller's name and use the name in the conversation, particularly at the conclusion of the call. Not only does this reduce possible confusion and error, but by asking for and using the caller's name, you communicate in a more personal manner.
6. If you must place the caller on hold (for a short time only) ask, "May I put you on hold while I look up your prescription?" In these circumstances, it is important that you do the following:
   a. Tell callers why you want to put them on hold.
   b. Ask if they would mind waiting a brief time or would prefer to call back (if appropriate).
   c. On returning to the telephone, say, "Thank you for waiting."
7. At the conclusion of the call, end it graciously (e.g., "Thank you for calling").
8. If possible, allow the caller to hang up first. This will allow the caller time to remember that extra request. It will also project in a subtle manner your sincere willingness to listen.

Besides receiving telephone calls, many times you must call physicians or other health care professionals to obtain additional information regarding a patient. The following suggestions may help make these calls more efficient.

1. Before you pick up the receiver, be sure you have any and all information related to the call before your conversation starts.
2. Before you pick up the receiver, determine with whom you need to speak in order to achieve your goal for calling.
3. Most importantly, before you pick up the receiver, ask yourself, "Is this call necessary?"
4. Identify yourself, your position, and the pharmacy first. Then, if it is not already provided to you, ask for the same information from the person who has answered your call.
5. After introducing yourself, state in clear, concise terms the reason for your

call. Be assertive! Do not begin by apologizing ("Sorry to bother you"). You have already decided that the call is necessary.

6. If the nature of your call dictates that it will exceed more than a couple of minutes, ask the person whether he or she has time to talk with you for a few minutes.
7. Conclude the conversation with a sincere "Thank you."

Summary

Gathering information from patients is a complex process that at times is difficult to master because it involves interactions between two persons. No two interactions are exactly the same, because the sequence of events and the people involved are never exactly the same. Interviews require different levels of flexibility based on the needs of the patient; they also require some type of structure to assure a time-efficient, clear exchange of information between you and the patient. In order to conduct a successful interview, certain communication skills need to be mastered. If the two parties are not communicating well, the entire interview process can break down, and the possibility of future positive interactions between the patient and pharmacist can be jeopardized. You must learn how to ask open-ended questions, to transmit information clearly, listen effectively, provide feedback, use silence, and develop rapport. Development of these skills takes time. In addition to using good communication skills, you must realize how to structure the interview. The type of environment, the type of approach, and how to start and how to end the interview are critical to the interview process.

The first step in improving this process is to realize that the effective use of these skills will lead to a more productive interview. You should evaluate each interview by asking such questions as "Did the patient appear to be relaxed and open?" or "Did I check to see whether the patient understood me correctly?" Such an analysis will reveal possible areas that need improvement.

The interview is a dynamic process that can always be improved. You cannot rest on previous successes, because many things in the process can be improved. At the same time, you should not worry about saying the wrong thing or putting your foot in your mouth. Most patients are forgiving, and relationships can be salvaged even after misunderstandings or ineffective communication. The key is to identify what went wrong, try to problem-solve and improve the communication as it progresses, and use more effective communication skills the next time you conduct an interview.

REVIEW QUESTIONS

1. **What are the critical components of an effective interview?**
2. **Why are people better senders of messages than receivers?**
3. **What are the differences between open-ended and closed-ended questions, and when should each be used?**
4. **What are five techniques that improve telephone productivity?**

REFERENCES

Beardsley RS, Johnson CA, Wise G. Privacy as a factor in patient counseling. *Journal of the American Pharmacists Association* NS17:366, 1977.

Bernstein L, Bernstein RS. *Interviewing: A Guide for Health Professionals*. New York, NY: Appleton-Century-Crofts, 1980.

Cipolle RJ, Strand LM, Morley PC. *Pharmaceutical Care Practice*. New York, NY: McGraw-Hill, 1998.

Gardner MG, Boyce RW, Herrier RN. *Pharmacist-Patient Consultation Program: An Interactive Approach to Verify Patient Understanding*. New York, NY: Pfizer, 1991.

Gardner MG, Boyce RW, Herrier RN. *Pharmacist-Patient Consultation Program, Unit 3: Counseling to Enhance Compliance*. New York, NY: Pfizer, 1995.

The Write Track: *Personal Health Teacher, Doctors & Designers*. Princeton, NJ: Bristol-Myers Squibb, 1997.

Wallerstein SL. Scaling clinical pain and pain relief. In Bromm B (ed.). *Pain Measurement in Man: Neurophysiological Correlates of Pain*. New York, NY: Elsevier, 1984.

Whooley MA, Avins AL, Miranda J, Browner WS. Case-finding instruments for depression: Two questions are as good as many. *Journal of General Internal Medicine* 12:439–445, 1997.

Willke RJ, Burke LB, Erickson P. Measuring treatment impact: A review of patient-reported outcomes and other efficacy endpoints in approved product labels. *Controlled Clinical Trials* 25:535–552, 2004.

RECOMMENDED READINGS

Krueger KP, Felkey BG, Berger BA. Improving adherence and persistence: A review and assessment of interventions and description of steps toward a national adherence initiative. *Journal of the American Pharmacists Association* 43:665, 2003.

Rollnick S, Mason P, Butler C. *Health Behavior Change: A Guide for Practitioners*. Edinburgh: Churchill Livingston, Robert Stevenson House, 1999.

CHAPTER

8

Helping Patients Manage Therapeutic Regimens

Overview

This chapter presents techniques to help patients manage drug therapy by building better patient understanding about their medication therapy and facilitating patient adherence to treatment regimens. Some of these techniques utilize specific communication skills discussed in previous chapters. Additional skills are described that help patients motivate themselves to make behavioral changes in the direction of improved health.

Introduction

A well-known physician once approached his colleagues with this admonition: "Keep watch also on the fault of patients which often makes them lie about taking of things prescribed." Hippocrates made this remark over 2,000 years ago! Unfortunately, concern about how patients actually use their prescribed medications continues to this day.

The terms "compliance," "adherence," and "concordance" have been used to describe the relationship between patient medication-taking behaviors and the regimens prescribed by providers. Sackett and Haynes (1976) defined compliance as the extent to which a person's behavior coincides with the medical advice given. This definition is in line with a more traditional patient–provider relationship in which providers told patients what to do and patients presumably did it (complied). The term "adherence" has largely replaced "compliance" and was intended to move away from the paternalistic view of patients as individuals who simply did as they were told. More recently, the term "concordance" has been used by some practitioners and researchers to acknowledge that patient medication use takes place in the context of the relationship between patients and providers. The Royal Pharmaceutical Society of Great Britain (1997) defined concordance as "an agreement reached after negotiation between a patient and health care professional that respects the beliefs and wishes of the patient in determining whether, when and how medicines are to be taken." Concordance obligates providers and patients to reach mutual decisions. This joint decision making requires a meaningful dialogue between patients and providers on medical options and patient preferences.

Lack of patient adherence to medication therapy remains a major health issue, according to the Institute of Medicine (IOM, 2001). The World Health Organization (2003) issued a report on adherence to long-term therapies summarizing what is known about rates of nonadherence for treatment of chronic conditions. The exact rate of adherence to medication regimens reviewed in this report varies from study to study since researchers in this area define and measure adherence differently. Some researchers use indirect methods of measuring adherence (interview patients and family members, have patients keep diaries) while others use more direct methods (assessing blood or urine levels of medication). However, regardless of definition and measurement, adherence rates are well below 100%. The consensus is that adherence rates for long-term therapies tend to be about 50%.

The exact cost of nonadherence is also unclear since it can affect so many aspects of medical care utilization and so many sources of direct and indirect costs associated with poorly controlled diseases. The costs also vary depending on the medical condition and type of therapy. In some conditions, costs are extremely high. For example, nonadherence has been found to be the primary predictor of rejection of transplanted organs, resulting in significant health care costs as well as increased suffering for patients (De Geest et al., 2001; Butler et al., 2004). Most nonadherences have negative effects on patient health which, in turn, can result in increased emergency room and physician visits, increased hospitalizations, decreased productivity in the work place, disability, and premature death.

Numerous reasons exist for why adherence is less than optimal. Some reasons are related to patients, some are related to health care providers, and others evolve from the health care delivery system. System issues include lack of insurance coverage, access to medications, and other economic concerns. Reasons for nonadherence to regimens include patient perception of medications and the perceived value of following treatment plans as prescribed. Patient perceptions of the severity of the illness, the value of treatment, and confidence in their own ability to adhere determine the likelihood of adherence (Johnson et al., 2003; Byrne et al., 2005; Godin et al., 2005). Patient beliefs in the positive outcomes of therapy as well as their confidence in their own ability to adhere are crucial. Many patients are afraid of taking medications, while some may rely too heavily on medications and take more than prescribed.

Simplified dosing regimens, particularly once a day dosing, have been found to be associated with higher rates of adherence (Iskedjian et al., 2002). In addition, higher levels of social support appear to consistently have a positive relationship to adherence (DiMatteo, 2004). A positive patient–provider relationship with a collaborative communication style has been found to be related to therapy adherence and to improved outcomes of treatment (Murphy et al., 2004; Maddigan et al., 2005; Lewis et al., 2006). Negative patient mood, including depression and anxiety, has been found to be associated with nonadherence in a number of disease states (Gonzalez et al., 2004; Gehi et al., 2005; Phillips et al., 2005). While certain variables have been found to be related to adherence, it is important to keep in mind that adherence is multidimensional with variability across different people as well as variability for an individual person in different situations, for different therapies, and for a specific therapy over time.

Before you are able to help a patient improve adherence to a treatment regimen, you must understand the underlying causes of the nonadherence in this particular patient. Nonadherence can be divided into two broad categories: unintentional (inadvertent) nonadherence and intentional nonadherence. Inadvertent nonadherence typically involves forgetting to take medications at prescribed times. Intentional nonadherence involves decisions a patient has made to alter a medication regimen or to discontinue drug therapy (permanently or temporarily). For example, a patient may decide to stop taking a medication due to an uncomfortable side effect or skip doses of a medication that should not be taken with alcohol before going to a party. As discussed in the following sections, you would use different approaches to resolving problems depending on the underlying cause of the nonadherence.

False Assumptions about Patient Understanding and Medication Adherence

As a pharmacist, you will be in a position to help patients avoid medication-related problems. In order to do this you must have a clear picture of what medications patients take, how they take them, and what their response to therapy has been, including both positive and negative perceptions. You should not make generalized assumptions nor take for granted that patients understand all aspects of their drug therapy before they get to the pharmacy. The following are common issues that should be kept in mind.

1. Do not assume that physicians have already discussed with patients the medications they prescribe. Makoul et al. (1995) found that physicians discussed instructions for taking a medication being prescribed during most encounters

(87%). However, only about half of the encounters included a discussion of the intended benefits of the medication. Possible side effects were discussed in 22% of encounters, and the patient's ability to follow the treatment plan was discussed in <5% of encounters.

2. Do not assume that patients understand all information provided. Even seemingly straightforward label directions like "take one tablet every six hours" are misinterpreted by a large percentage of patients (Hanchak et al., 1996). For patients, every 6 hours is often interpreted to mean that they are supposed to take doses only during waking hours and thus take only three doses a day. Number of doses per day and recommended spacing of doses, along with the minimum safe spacing of doses, should be understood by patients. Written information for a variety of medications advises: "If you miss a dose, take it as soon as you can. If it is too close to the next dose, skip the dose. Do not double up on doses." Such advice is not specific enough unless you give information on how close is "too close" in the spacing of doses for any particular medication.
3. Do not assume that if patients understand what is required, they will be able to take the medication correctly. Understanding of regimen demands is necessary but not sufficient to assure adherence. Implementing a new medication regimen requires a change in behavior, which is often difficult.
4. Do not assume that when patients do not take their medications correctly that they "don't care," "aren't motivated," "lack intelligence," or "can't remember." These assumptions prevent you from focusing on the real problems causing nonadherence. Many patients want to take their medications correctly but are not able to manage this due to a variety of reasons that will be discussed later in this chapter.
5. Do not assume that once patients start taking their medications correctly, they will continue to take them correctly in the future. You need to assess medication use and reinforce key messages during subsequent patient counseling sessions. Often patients adhere to regimens while health care providers monitor adherence closely but lapse into nonadherence as provider attention and reinforcement decrease (Patel et al., 2005). The challenge is to help motivate patients to take their medications correctly when there is no apparent harm that they can detect from not doing so.
6. Do not assume that physicians routinely monitor patient medication use and will thus intervene if problems exist. Because many patients visit multiple physicians, physician office records are often incomplete. In addition, physicians vary greatly in their skills in assessing patient adherence (Sherman et al., 2000).
7. Do not assume that if patients are having problems, they will ask direct questions or volunteer information. Avoid being lulled into complacency by thinking that if patients have problems they will contact you. This assumption ignores the fact that patients may be embarrassed to admit having problems or may not even realize they have a problem. You must initiate interaction by asking the open-ended questions discussed in earlier chapters.

Techniques to Improve Patient Understanding

Once you have assessed patient understanding of medications, you can enhance patient adherence by filling in the information gaps with easy-to-understand language. This allows you to target your education to patient needs. The following strategies can assist in your patient education efforts.

1. Emphasize key points. Telling patients beforehand "This is very important" helps them remember what follows.
2. Give reasons for key advice. For example, with an antibiotic prescription, tell why it is necessary to continue medication use even though symptoms have disappeared. Patients should understand the reasons behind what you and the physician are instructing them. When reasons for advice are provided, patients are more likely to perceive the advice as important.
3. Give definite, concrete, explicit instructions. Any information that patients can mentally picture is more easily remembered. Use visual aids, photographs, or demonstrations. When patients are given specific, easy-to-understand instructions, they tend to regard this advice as more important than when advice is given in general terms.
4. Provide key information at the beginning and end of the interaction. Patients concentrate on the initial information given and also remember the last items discussed.
5. End the encounter by giving patients the opportunity to provide feedback about what they learned. You should ask patients to summarize critical points of information so that you can make sure you communicated clearly and patients understand accurately. If patients do not understand, this is not a reflection on them but rather an indication that you must do a better job in communication and educational efforts.

Supplementing oral instructions with written information is an essential part of patient counseling. Refer to advice in the written information as you counsel patients. Highlighting written material and explaining the importance of particular pieces of advice can serve as a guide for you in structuring the counseling session and provide a point of reference for patients when they read the material. Selecting the appropriate written information is crucial since the quality and quantity of material are quite varied. The material must be comprehensive and yet presented in an interesting and easy-to-read form.

Before using written material, assess the level of literacy required to read and understand the information. Low health literacy, which includes deficiencies in both reading skill and ability to accurately interpret health advice, is associated with poor understanding of instructions, increased nonadherence, and poorer health outcomes (AHRQ, 2005). A reading level of fifth to seventh grade will ensure readability by the majority of adults (Doak et al., 1996). In order to achieve a reading level that those with marginal literacy will understand, use short words, short sentences, and words that are written in lay rather than medical language. An option for evaluating the level of readability exists in Microsoft Word (see Box 8.1).

BOX 8.1 Using the Readability Option in Microsoft Word

To set up program in Microsoft Word 2010:

1. Click the **File** tab, and then click **Options**.
2. Click Proofing.
3. Under **When correcting spelling and grammar in Word,** make sure **Check grammar with spelling** is selected.
4. Select **Show readability statistics**.
5. After you enable this feature, open a file that you want to check, and *check the spelling and skip line before starting the next line.*

To set up program in Microsoft Word 2007:

1. Click the **Microsoft Office Button**, and then click **Word Options**.
2. Click **Proofing**.
3. Make sure **Check grammar with spelling** is selected.
4. Under **When correcting grammar in Word**, select **Show readability statistics**.

To set up program in previous versions of Microsoft Word:

1. Clink on **Tools** in the top menu.
2. Select **Options**.
3. Select **Spelling & Grammar**.
4. Select the **Show readability statistics** box from the bottom of the list.

Even with easy-to-read written materials, you must still verify that the information is understood by an individual patient. Assessment of a patient's ability to read and understand key written instructions is required. Asking patients to read the medication label instructions and describe how they intend to take the medication is one strategy to get an initial impression of reading ability and health literacy. Reluctance to fill out forms without "taking them home" may be a cue that the patient has literacy problems. Tell a patient "Some of the information in these medication leaflets I give you can be hard to understand. How much trouble have you had in the past understanding information in a leaflet like this?" This may encourage patients to tell you about difficulties they encounter with written information. Inability to read and interpret label directions, while possibly pointing to low health literacy, could also be caused by other problems such as visual or cognitive impairments. Once difficulty reading or understanding is identified, the underlying cause of the problem must still be accurately defined.

Techniques to Establish New Behaviors

A number of simple suggestions from you when patients are beginning a new regimen can help get them started on the right track. These strategies can

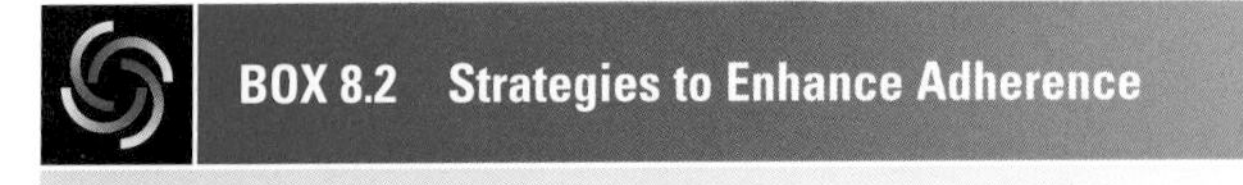

BOX 8.2 Strategies to Enhance Adherence

- Integrate new behaviors into patient lifestyle
- Provide or suggest compliance or reminder aids
- Suggest patient self-monitoring
- Monitor use on an ongoing basis
- Refer patients when necessary

make it easier for patients to establish a new routine of taking medications. See Box 8.2.

1. Help patients identify ways to integrate new behaviors with current habits. This strategy is known as "tailoring" of regimens. It is hard for anyone to establish new behaviors. Linking new behaviors (taking a medication) to habitual behaviors, such as brushing teeth before going to bed, preparing dinner, or dressing for work, helps immensely in establishing a new behavior. Other strategies include setting alarms, posting reminder notes in obvious places such as the bathroom mirror or the refrigerator, and storing medications where they will be seen at the time they are to be taken. Having a reminder system in place "cues" patients to take the medication at the right times (Figure 8-1).

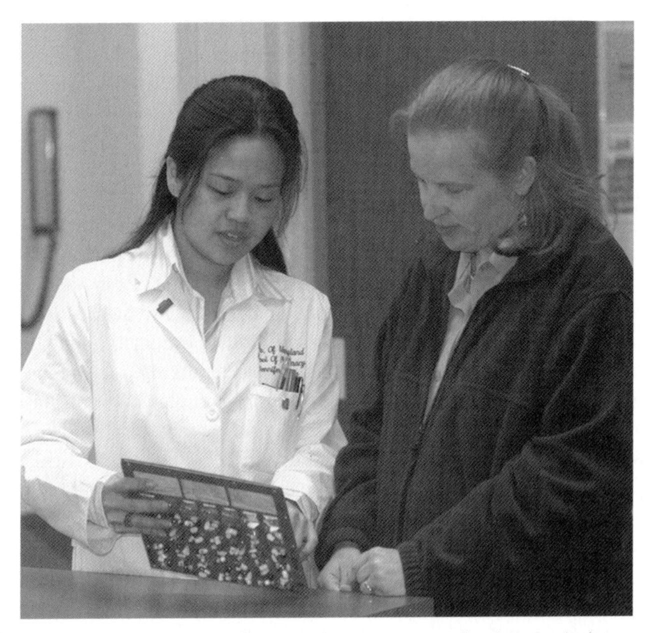

FIGURE 8-1. Pharmacist showing patient how to use medication reminder system.

2. Provide appropriate adherence aids. Individualized medication packaging for daily or weekly doses seems to work for some patients (Smith, 1989; Connor et al., 2004). Alarms on cell phones and other devices can be programmed to signal when medication doses are to be taken. Some people record medications on their personal calendars (e.g., their Google calendars).
3. Suggest ways to self-monitor. One simple way to help patients monitor medication taking is to suggest that they use a medication diary or calendar on which to record their medication use. This helps not only problems of forgetting to take medication but also the problem of forgetting whether a dose has been taken 10 minutes ago or not. Other monitoring can involve treatment effects. Seeing differences in physiological parameters can be a strong reinforcement for continuing to take medications. Thus, patients can monitor their response to treatment, such as by taking their own blood pressure or testing their blood glucose levels. Understanding the goals of therapy and having a way to judge their own progress helps patients establish and maintain adherent behaviors.
4. Monitor medication use. With chronic care medications, you should monitor adherence frequently and assess patient perception of effectiveness and problems encountered. You should review prescription records for potential problems, such as patterns of late refills. Refill reminder software systems are available to generate reports and to implement reminder systems, such as creating reminder mailings when refills are due. Many pharmacists also call patients to see how they are taking the medication and responding to therapy after they start on a new prescription.
5. Make proper referrals. In cases involving lack of access to care, you will want to refer patients to appropriate social service agencies, such as government programs for low-income patients. Barriers to proper adherence can obviously include patients' inability to obtain needed medications. Information on sources of financial help is found on websites such as *www.needymeds.com* and *www.medicare.gov* (for information on Medicare Part D plans).

Techniques to Facilitate Behavior Change

As we said earlier, behavior change is difficult. Anyone who has tried to implement a new exercise regimen, stop smoking, change diet, floss teeth daily, eat five servings of fruits and vegetables a day, or begin a new medication regimen can testify to the difficulties involved. It is difficult to establish a new habit such as beginning a medication regimen, to change old habits such as overeating, and to stop existing habits such as smoking. The more complex and multifaceted the behavior change required, the more difficult the change will be. For chronic diseases such as diabetes, the changes prescribed by health providers involve establishing new behaviors (drug therapy and daily blood glucose monitoring), changing old habits (diet and exercise), and ceasing other behaviors (drinking alcohol). In addition to the distress of discovering that you have a chronic disease, the sheer number of changes you are asked to make can seem overwhelming.

Individuals who are forced to change habits or start long-term therapy often are ambivalent about the changes they are asked to make. They are usually able to see the benefits of changing their behaviors, but they also have a reinforcement history and hold existing beliefs that support their current habits. There are likely to be downsides or perceived costs associated with both changing behaviors and maintaining the status quo. The result is ambivalence. Ambivalence regarding changing behavior exists when patients feel they want to make changes to improve their health but, at the same time, they resent changing behaviors they have found comfortable in the past. They thus feel contradictory feelings. Ambivalence is a state of contradictory emotions at the same time related to the same situation. The specific contradictory emotions involved can be quite varied. Persons can be defiant and angry about pressures to change, but also feel remorse about the costs and consequences of not changing (a frequent conflict in substance abuse situations). They can move between blaming others and being consumed by guilt, between denial and acceptance of the need to change. Such a conflict is called an "approach-avoidance" conflict whereby the person vacillates between indulging in and resisting the old behavior. In the most extreme situations, patients can vacillate between being hopeful about the future and feeling hopeless, with accompanying feelings of depression and despair. The ambivalence does not mean patients are unwilling to change, but they feel conflicted between wanting to change and wanting to stay the same. Your goal here is to help patients move from being ambivalent to being willing to begin the process of change.

Theoretical Foundations Supporting Behavior Change

Miller and Rollnick (2002) developed a conceptual foundation and intervention strategies, known as Motivational Interviewing, to help people make changes in the direction of better health. They identified three components of motivation to change: (a) willingness, which is indicated by the amount of discrepancy patients perceive between current health status and goals they have for themselves, (b) perceived ability or the amount of self-confidence patients feel in their ability to initiate and maintain behavioral change (also known as self-efficacy), and (c) readiness, which is related to how high a priority is given to these behavioral changes. Often patients will want to delay a commitment to initiate change because other stressors in their lives make changing their own behaviors seem daunting.

Motivational Interviewing focuses on the process of communication between patient and provider. It incorporates many of the relationship-building principles and techniques of Carl Rogers (1951, 1961), which were discussed in Chapter 5. Empathic understanding is a core skill in both approaches. Rogers emphasized that empathic understanding is a core condition of a helping relationship because it facilitates the patient's own problem-solving ability. Empathic understanding from a provider frees patients from the fear that they are being judged because of their behavior. This "safe environment" allows patients to trust providers enough to confide in them the truth about the struggles they face in efforts to change. Rogers' theory is said to be client- or patient-centered because the crucial decision to change is seen to reside in the patient. Providers can only assist a patient in making informed decisions that are consistent with the patient's own goals. Motivational Interviewing, while patient-centered in the Rogerian sense, is more direct in encouraging change in a particular direction that is consistent with the goals of improved health. The pharmacist would help patients resolve feelings of ambivalence, which would move them toward initiating change. The ambivalence appears as patients want to change because of their knowledge that it is important for improved health yet at the same time feel comfortable with their old, familiar patterns of behavior.

Motivational Interviewing also incorporates constructs and techniques associated with a social cognitive framework. According to the social cognitive theory of Albert Bandura (1986), behavior change requires that an individual believe that (a) "engaging in a particular behavior change will lead to an outcome I desire" (outcome expectancy) and (b) "I am capable of carrying out the behavior change" (self-efficacy expectancy). Outcome beliefs are persuasive. If patients do not believe taking antihypertensive medications will really affect their quality of life or longevity, they will probably not be willing to initiate treatment. If smokers believe the research linking smoking and premature death is exaggerated or somehow does not apply to them personally (think of the patient whose father smoked heavily his whole life and lived to be 90), they are unlikely to stop smoking. In addition to believing the change of behavior is linked to positive health outcomes, patients must perceive that they are capable of initiating and maintaining the change.

Self-efficacy in a medication adherence framework is a person's confidence that he or she can adhere to a regimen even in situations that make it difficult to do so. For use of a metered dose inhaler (MDI) for albuterol in treatment of asthma, self-efficacy may involve confidence in ability to use the MDI at a party or in a classroom if the need arises. For abstinence from alcohol, self-efficacy may involve confidence in ability to adhere to abstinence even at a holiday party, which is a high-risk situation. Confidence in ability to overcome temptations to relapse even in high-risk situations is a key component of self-efficacy beliefs. If patients have tried and failed to maintain changes in the past, this can result in doubts about their own self-efficacy. It is important to keep in mind that most persons who are successful in maintaining changes are able to do so in spite of the fact that they made previous attempts that failed. Successful change of behavior, such as a permanent cessation of smoking, is unlikely to take place on the first attempt the person makes to quit smoking. Persistence, deciding to try one more time, is key to successful behavior change. Finding other people who can serve as role models for maintenance of change can be effective, which is often the benefit of support groups or 12-step programs such as Alcoholics Anonymous.

In addition, Motivational Interviewing builds upon a foundation consistent with the Transtheoretical Model of Change. The Transtheoretical Model of Change (Prochaska and DiClemente, 1982) differs from client-centered therapy and a social cognitive perspective by focusing on the stages a person goes through in making decisions to change their behavior. The importance of empathy, self-efficacy, and outcome expectancies continue throughout the transition from one stage to another. Behavior change is seen as a process that continues over time rather than as a defining moment or single event. The stages conceptualized by the model are described in the following sections See Box 8.3.

STAGE 1: PRECONTEMPLATION

In this stage, persons do not intend to change their behavior or implement new behaviors. They may be uninformed about the benefits of change or may minimize the risks to their health of continuing their current practices. Interventions with persons who are not motivated to change must focus on getting them to *think about* changing habits, to consider information or evidence provided, or to begin to consider the pros and cons of behavior change. Brief, simple advice with reasons can be given in a nonjudgmental or nondictatorial way. From then on, you must listen to patients and understand concerns expressed. Confronting reluctant patients is likely to begin a process of resistance to change rather than helping to facilitate change.

STAGE 2: CONTEMPLATION

The contemplation stage is one where individuals are "thinking about" changing their behavior—not immediately but within the next 6 months or so. They believe in the benefits of change but also see the personal costs or challenges involved. They feel ambivalent.

Interventions at this stage can best be focused on getting patients to describe the "pros" to making changes and to explore what might help them overcome barriers they perceive. It is best to have patients make the arguments themselves on the desirable aspects of initiating a change in behavior. If a patient says he knows it would improve his health if he stopped smoking, but he is "not ready" to quit immediately, asking how he will know when it is the right time can help the planning process without sounding argumentative. Helping patients define the goals they have for their own health and gently identifying discrepancies between goals and behavior can facilitate change. Above all, empathy and encouragement when patients express confidence in themselves helps to maintain positive patient–pharmacist relationships and increase patient motivation and self-confidence to change.

STAGE 3: PREPARATION

In the preparation stage, the individual is ready to implement a change program or initiate a new regimen almost immediately (within a month). These individuals have reached a decision in favor of change. Reinforcement from you and others can help them carry out these decisions. In addition, teaching patients strategies to help them be successful in initiating change is important. Helping patients define "right-sized" goals that they feel confident they can achieve is particularly valuable. Patients can be helped to view change as a process rather than an event. Taking small steps with successive advancements toward the ultimate goal may be a reasonable approach to take with some behavioral changes. Once change is initiated, patients should have realistic expectations about the challenges ahead but also feel capable of meeting the goals they set. For some changes, patients may need information on strategies specific to the changes they are making (e.g., special diets). In addition, patients may be helped by referrals to specialized sources of assistance (e.g., dieticians, counseling services).

STAGE 4: ACTION

The action stage is the initial period in changing a behavior. This stage is thought to incorporate the first 6 months. During this initial period of change, the desire to go back to old habits makes the potential to relapse of concern. You can use some of the strategies identified in the "Principles and Strategies" section below to help "inoculate" against relapse. In addition, continued positive reinforcement for the small successes, for the "progress" being made in reaching goals, is extremely helpful. Attention should be given to the triumphs experienced rather than only to the problems encountered and the slips that occur.

STAGE 5: MAINTENANCE

In the maintenance stage, relapse can continue to be of concern but persons can often continue with the new habits without constant vigilance against relapse. The new behaviors have become more integrated into lifestyles and routines. Patients gain more confidence in their abilities to maintain changes. However, for certain changes, such as abstinence from addictive substances, dangers of relapse continue indefinitely.

BOX 8.3 Stages of Change

Stage	Defining Characteristics	Communication Approaches
Precontemplation	Unwillingness to change	Raise awareness of problem
	Lack recognition of problem	Provide information
	Deny seriousness of risks	Convey empathy
		Encourage "thinking about"
		Express willingness to help
		Avoid arguing

Box 8.3 cont.

Contemplation	"Thinking about" change	Encourage patient to list pros and cons
	Aware of consequences of inaction	Elicit reasons in favor of change
	Willing to change within 6 months	Reinforce positive statements
		Acknowledge ambivalence
		Show empathy
		Identify discrepancy between goals and behavior
		Encourage small steps
Preparation	Commitment to change (<1 month)	Help patient formulate specific plan
	Benefits seen to outweigh costs	Tailor plan to patient needs
		Ask about barriers to change
		Discuss ways to overcome barriers
		Provide information and referrals as needed
Action	Change is initiated	Provide positive reinforcement
	Challenges experienced	Focus on benefits of change
	Effort to maintain resolve	Discuss strategies to prevent relapse
		Discuss "slips" vs. "relapse"
Maintenance	Change established (>6 months)	Continue reinforcement for success
	Change incorporated into lifestyle	Assist in problem solving in case of a lapse
	Focus is on avoiding relapse	

In any stage, regression to an earlier stage can occur. In fact, for many key changes, including diet, exercise, smoking, alcohol consumption, and medication adherence, relapse at some point in the change process should be considered the norm rather than an unexpected aberration. Helping patients identify temptations to relapse and strategies to cope effectively with temptations is an important aspect of promoting behavior change.

BOX 8.4 Motivating Patients to Change

- Express empathy
- Develop discrepancy
- Roll with resistance
- Support self-efficacy
- Elicit and reinforce "change talk"

Applying Motivational Interviewing Principles and Strategies

Motivational Interviewing focuses on techniques to help motivate patients to move through the stages of change. Using Motivational Interviewing at the depth described by Miller and Rollnick (2002) probably requires specialized training as well as adequate time to devote to an individual patient. However, the qualities of a helping relationship and techniques applied in Motivational Interviewing can be helpful in even brief encounters with patients (Miller and Rollnick, 2002). Some of the principles and techniques of Motivational Interviewing are summarized below in Box 8.4.

EXPRESS EMPATHY

Convey to patients that you understand the difficulty of change. You are not judgmental even when patients are unwilling to begin or unable to maintain changes. Reflective listening and acceptance of patient feelings and struggles are core conditions for the helping relationship (Rogers, 1951, 1961). It is especially helpful to convey understanding of the ambivalence that is inevitable in the change process. Pressuring patients to change increases resistance rather than helping to initiate and maintain change (see Case Study 8.1).

CASE STUDY 8.1

Your patient is a 50-year-old woman who has had type 2 diabetes for 1 year. She is 5′2″, says she weighs 220 pounds, and reports her self-monitored glucose to be "about" 200. Her last lab report shows HbA1c to be 9.

Patient: I know that my diabetes is a serious problem. I have read that diabetes can kill you or make you go blind. I certainly want to stick around to see my grandkids grow up.

Pharmacist: Your grandchildren are important to you and you want to be there for them. [Empathic response]

Patient: Absolutely. It's just so hard to do everything—diet, exercise, take medications, test my blood.

Pharmacist: So even though you want to make changes, you feel overwhelmed. [Empathy for ambivalent feelings.]

CASE STUDY 8.2

Patient: I know I have to get my blood sugar down. And I really want to lose weight. But I just can't stick to that diet. I love fried chicken and biscuits and gravy and sweets too much to cut them out.

Pharmacist: It sounds like you resent having to cut down on the foods you love. But, it also sounds as if you would like to lose weight and get your blood sugar levels down.

Patient: I would like to lose weight. I know it is not good for me to be so overweight.

Pharmacist: So you have the goal of losing weight but you know that the foods you eat are preventing you from reaching your goal. [Reflection of discrepancy between goals and current behaviors]

DEVELOP DISCREPANCY

Help patients identify the discrepancy that exists between their current behaviors and their stated values or goals. Let patients present the arguments in favor of change. As Miller and Rollnick (2002) note, "People are often more persuaded by what they hear themselves say than by what other people tell them" (p. 39) (see Case Study 8.2)

ROLL WITH RESISTANCE

Patient resistance to suggested changes is often exacerbated by the communication style of the pharmacist. Arguing with patients about the necessity of behavioral change may cause them to argue the other side (remember, they feel ambivalent) and point out why change is not feasible right now. Resistance will also be increased if you seem to be blaming patients for not "adhering" to regimen demands, seem to be in a hurry for patients to make progress, or imply that you know better than patients how to proceed. You must accept the fact that decisions to change inevitably come from patients. Acknowledge to patients that their ambivalence and reluctance to change are understandable. Reinforce the patient's role as the key problem-solver. Have patients identify ways to meet goals they have articulated. If you see patients arguing with you, it is time to change the way you are responding (see Case Study 8.3).

In any case, avoid arguing with your patient. You want to stay on the patient's side, and arguing can make patients feel defensive. Rather than moving toward changing their behaviors, they may instead stop telling you the truth about the problems they have in adhering to medical recommendations (see Case Study 8.4).

CASE STUDY 8.3

Diabetic patient: I'm tired of everyone telling me I should lose weight. My kids are always on me about following my diet.

Pharmacist: You sound discouraged with the diet and annoyed that everyone is giving you advice.

Patient: I am discouraged. Of course I want to lose weight, but it is not easy.

Pharmacist: What do you think you can do to help reach your goal?

Patient: I don't know. I just hate giving up all the foods I love.

Pharmacist: Maybe you could start with a smaller step. Are you ready to consider making small changes in your diet and see how that goes? Sometimes even a small change can help control your diabetes.

Patient: I don't know.

Pharmacist: You may not be ready to change your eating habits right now. If you decide you would like to try making some changes, there is a dietician I know who has helped other diabetic people lose weight. You may want to schedule a time to talk to her at some point.

CASE STUDY 8.4

Diabetic patient: I wish people would quit nagging me about my diet.

Pharmacist: You're right. It really is up to you whether or not you change your eating habits.

Patient: I know my kids mean well.

Pharmacist: So you think your kids nag because they are worried about your health?

Patient: Everyone in my family is overweight. It is in my genes.

Pharmacist: There is some evidence of a genetic tendency to be overweight. Diabetics who have been heavy all their lives but do lose weight often try many different strategies until they find something that works for them.

SUPPORT SELF-EFFICACY

Reinforce patient statements that reflect positive attitudes and optimism about ability to change. Offer options for patients to consider. Encourage patients to talk with others who have overcome obstacles to change and have discovered strategies that worked for them. Observing how others like themselves overcome

CASE STUDY 8.5

Pharmacist: What have you tried before that has been successful in changing diet or exercise habits?

Patient: I did start a diet and exercise program when I first found out I was diabetic. I lost 25 pounds. But I only stuck with it for 3 months.

Pharmacist: Twenty-five pounds is a lot. Those 3 months show you can be successful. We can work on strategies for maintaining the changes for longer if you are ready to do that. How were you able to make the changes that you made the last time?

challenges can be a powerful way of learning (Bandura, 1986). This is one reason support groups can be helpful to some individuals. However, the most important learning comes from one's own "mastery" experiences where one makes changes in line with goals. This is why it is so important to help patients define small steps for change that they feel confident they can achieve. In this way they can experience success, thus increasing their sense of self-efficacy and confidence in their ability to change. They can, step by step, come ever closer to meeting their goals (see Case Study 8.5).

Commonly used Motivational Interviewing questions allow assessment of the perceived importance of behavior change and perceived confidence in making the change (Miller and Rollnick, 2002). Examples of questions include: "How important would you say it is for you to change your eating habits? On a scale from zero to 10 where zero is not important and 10 is extremely important, where would you say you are?" and "How confident would you say you are that, if you decided to change your eating habits, you could do it?" If a patient says he is a "6" on the importance ruler, the pharmacist might ask "Why did you say 6 instead of 2 or 3?" as a way to focus attention on the positive expectations that are present. A further question may be "What would it take to get you to an 8 or 9?" as a means of identifying perceived barriers that will have to be overcome before change will occur.

ELICIT AND REINFORCE "CHANGE TALK"

Encourage patients to take action. Discuss a range of steps that could be taken to get closer to health goals rather than promoting "all or none" thinking for complex changes. Helping patients choose right-sized steps that they feel confident they can meet will build confidence in their abilities to manage their conditions. Praise ideas patients have to address their own problems. Offer information on change strategies or sources of help if patients wish for your suggestions. Be familiar with referral sources so you are able to provide accurate information on sources of help, along with contact persons to facilitate referrals.

IMPLEMENT "RELAPSE PREVENTION" PROGRAM

For many of us, the challenge is not in changing behavior but in maintaining the changes we make. Mark Twain reportedly said, "It's easy to stop smoking. I've done it hundreds of times." In fact, few people are able to maintain change the first time they try. A number of factors have been found to be related to relapse or backsliding into old patterns of behavior (Prochaska et al., 1994; Marlatt et al., 2002). These include:

1. Emotional distress, particularly anxiety, depression, worry, boredom, and interpersonal conflict
2. Social pressure
3. Guilt and self-blame for lapses or one-time slips
4. Overconfidence ("I can smoke one cigarette and stop again")
5. Frequent temptation (meeting the same drinking buddies after work at a bar, keeping a pack of cigarettes on hand to prove one can resist)
6. Desire for immediate gratification ("I deserve a drink after a hard day," "Changing should not be this hard," "It takes too long to notice weight change")

To help patients prevent relapse—a more permanent regression to an unhealthy behavior pattern—the following steps are recommended See Box 8.5:

1. Help patients understand the critical difference between a "slip" or "lapse" (having a bowl of ice cream) and "relapse" (abandoning the goal of reducing fat and calorie intake). Lapses are not "failures" and can often be understood in terms of response to a negative emotion (eating when feeling under stress) or being in a situation that presents strong temptation (being at a holiday party). People who think of a lapse as a personal failure ("I have no willpower") are more likely to slip from a "lapse" into a "relapse" than are those who think of a lapse as a temporary inability to cope with a specific situation.
2. Help patients identify the high-risk situations in which they are most vulnerable. This helps them anticipate situations that are likely to be difficult for them. Encourage patients, then, to mentally rehearse how they will handle these situations.
3. Lapses should be seen as learning experiences. Encourage patients to identify what might help them to cope with a similar situation in the future. This may involve enlisting friends to provide support. For complex behavioral change regimens, such as treatment of diabetes, support groups can be helpful for individuals who lack a supportive social network.
4. If patients lapse, help them have a plan in place ahead of time to go back to the new behavioral regimen without feeling guilty. The desire to revert to old habits will continue, and the key is to have a plan to help maintain new habits in spite of these desires. This plan may involve reviewing the reasons why the behavior change was made in the first place, to remind oneself of the health goals that were behind the decision. The plan may also involve changing one's specific thoughts about the lapse. For example, rather than thinking "I'm a failure. I don't have the willpower to maintain an exercise program," think more

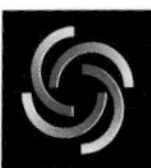

BOX 8.5 Preventing and Coping with Relapses

- Help patients understand the difference between a lapse and relapse
- Help patients identify the high-risk situations in which they are most vulnerable to lapsing into old habits
- Help patients identify what might help them to cope with a similar situation in the future
- Help patients have a plan in place ahead of time to go back to the new behavior without feeling guilty
- Help patients recommit to goals of change
- For patients who are hindered by chronic or severe emotional distress, refer to physicians or a mental health professional

rational thoughts such as: "I did not do my exercise routine as planned yesterday. However, I still want to reach my long-term goal of improved cardiovascular health. Yesterday I slipped up by not leaving work in time and getting caught in traffic. I am going to get back in the exercise program today. If I set my watch alarm, maybe I won't lose track of time. I am going to leave work regardless of how busy I am. It is the only way I will meet my fitness goal."

Encourage thinking that is about problem solving rather than self-blame or regret. A recommitment to goals of change must be made on an ongoing basis throughout the change process. For patients who are hindered by chronic or severe emotional distress, referral to their physicians or a mental health professional is indicated.

Summary

Adherence to medication regimens can be improved by enhancing patient understanding about the medication and by facilitating the patient's motivation to take the medication appropriately. You must assess patient knowledge about medications, educate patients regarding essential information, assess medication-taking behaviors, and provide strategies to change behaviors that are at variance with desired health outcomes.

Communication to achieve better outcomes is complex. Expecting patients to easily change their behaviors because providers tell them to do so is naive. Behavior change is difficult, and relapse to old, unhealthy habits is common. Assessing patient motivation to adhere to health advice can identify perceived barriers to taking prescribed medication. Helping patients to maintain changes they have made to improve their health requires ongoing attention and reinforcement from you. Case Study 8.6 demonstrates one approach to counseling a patient using a variety of previously discussed communication techniques to enhance patient understanding and adherence.

CASE STUDY 8.6

Counseling a Patient with a New Prescription

This case illustrates how the various components of counseling could be applied to a clinical scenario. The suggested dialogue is provided on the left for each of the critical components of the counseling process on the right. The rationale for using specific dialogue is also provided for the various segments.

Ms. Burris is a 45-year-old woman who comes to pick up a new Rx for Lipitor 40 mg tablets to be taken one tablet once daily. A few years ago Dr. Perkins helped her select a multivitamin when she complained of general fatigue and it seemed to help, along with her joining a lunchtime walking club. She has been a regular patient but is not currently taking any other chronic therapies.

Conversation	Analysis
Dr. Perkins: Good morning, are you Ms. Burris?	Identify patient by name.
Ms. Burris: Yes, I'm Ms. Burris.	Introduce yourself by name.
Dr. Perkins: Great, I'm Dr. Perkins, the pharmacist who filled your prescription from your physician, Dr. Johnson.	Identify prescriber by name.
If it is all right with you, I'd like to take a few minutes to discuss your Lipitor prescription with you. This should help prevent problems when you get home and start taking this medication.	Get patient consent. Establish purpose, importance, and length of counseling.
Ms. Burris: That's fine.	
Dr. Perkins: Before we get started, I need to identify what medications you are allergic to.	Identify medication allergies.
Ms. Burris: None.	
Dr. Perkins: What other prescription medications are you currently taking?	Identify other prescription medications being used.
Ms. Burris: None.	
Dr. Perkins: What nonprescription medications are you taking?	Identify OTC products used.

Case Study 8.6, cont.

Ms. Burris: None.	
Dr. Perkins: What herbals, vitamins, or supplements are you taking?	Identify other agents used.
Ms. Burris: None.	

Rationale: It is important to correctly identify your patient before providing the medication and data. If someone arrives to claim a prescription for a patient, he or she must provide verification of his or her relationship to the patient. It is prudent to record the name of the person who received the prescription(s) and his or her relationship to the patient, along with a sentence about the information provided on your patient's profile or on the back of the original prescription.

Conversation	**Analysis**
Dr. Perkins: This is what your medication looks like [opens prescription vial]. It is Lipitor 40 mg, also known as atorvastatin. Have you taken this medication previously?	State medication name and dose. State generic name when appropriate. Determine history of use.
Ms. Burris: No, I never have.	
Dr. Perkins: Please tell me, what did Dr. Johnson tell you this medication was for?	Ask open-ended question: indication for use.
Ms. Burris: It's going to lower my cholesterol.	
Dr. Perkins: That's right. Along with changes in your diet, this medication will help your high cholesterol.	Verify current medical condition.
Explain indication for use.	
Ms. Burris: How does it do that?	
Dr. Perkins: Lipitor essentially blocks an enzyme necessary to produce "bad" cholesterol (called LDL or low-density lipoprotein). It can also increase levels of "good" cholesterol (called HDL or high-density lipoprotein). These actions lower the risk of heart attacks.	Explain how the medication works in layman's terms.

Case Study 8.6, cont.

Rationale: Hold the medication container label toward Ms. Burris, point at the label, and state the name of the medication and the label directions. Avoid the use of technical terms and phrases. Remember to use good "attending behaviors," i.e., standing or sitting at the same level as the patient, leaning forward, using good eye contact, nodding, and giving verbal encouragement appropriately.

Conversation	Analysis
Dr. Perkins: How have you been told to take this medication?	Ask open-ended question: how to use
Ms. Burris: Just once a day, I guess.	
Dr. Perkins: Yes. It is best to take it the same time each day. You can take it with or without food. You will be taking it for a long time, until Dr. Johnson tells you differently.	State schedule. State duration of use.
Sometimes it is difficult to take a new medication exactly as prescribed. Have you had difficulty taking other medications in the past?	Probe for adherence problems.
Ms. Burris: Sometimes.	
Dr. Perkins: What caused the difficulty?	Probe for reasons for adherence problems.
Ms. Burris: It was sometimes hard to remember to take medicine. I would get busy and forget.	
Dr. Perkins: It may be best to take Lipitor around an activity you do every day at the same time, such as at dinner or before going to bed. Some patients benefit from using a Saturday through Sunday weekly pill box. If you miss a dose, take it immediately after you realize it, unless you have <12 hours before your next dose. Take the next dose at your regular time. Store Lipitor in a cool, dry place.	Recommend strategies to enhance adherence. Instruct on how to handle a missed dose. Explain special storage instructions.

Rationale: Hold the container so that Ms. Burris can see the labeled area, and point to and explain how to take the medication.

Case Study 8.6, cont.

Conversation	Analysis
Dr. Perkins: What did Dr. Johnson tell you to expect from this medication? (*Ms. Burris looks confused.*) How do you think it will make you feel?	Ask open-ended question regarding positive effects of drug.
Ms. Burris: I don't know. How?	
Dr. Perkins: You probably won't feel any differently and won't be able to tell whether the drug is actually working or not. What did Dr. Johnson say he would do to make sure your medicine is working for you?	Explain expected outcome. Explain how to monitor for efficacy.
Ms. Burris: He said I would go back in a month to have my blood tested. Then he said he would check it every 3 months.	
Dr. Perkins: What did he tell you about the cholesterol levels you should have after you have taken Lipitor for a while?	
Ms. Burris: He told me some numbers but I don't remember what they were.	
Dr. Perkins: You might want to discuss this with him when you go in next month. It is especially important to see the "bad" cholesterol—LDL—go down.	

Rationale: Patients should know how to monitor themselves to see how the drug is working, which helps adherence. Unfortunately, patients don't feel any differently when taking some medications, and they should know that they will not be able to tell how well the drug is working based on their own symptoms or perceptions.

Conversation	Analysis
Dr. Perkins: I realize there is a lot of information out there about Lipitor thanks to advertisements. What have you heard about the side effects or precautions with Lipitor?	Ask open-ended question regarding side effects of drug.
Ms. Burris: Nothing really, I haven't paid much attention.	Explain warnings or precautions.

Case Study 8.6, cont.

Dr. Perkins: I will send you home with this written information that you can refer to. As you can see on this material, there are just a few key precautions. First, if you have a history of problems with your liver, you should not take it. In fact, Dr. Johnson will be testing your liver about every 6 months to make sure that it is okay. Second, it should not be taken by women who are nursing, pregnant, or may want to be pregnant. Probably the most important side effect is muscle weakness. If you feel any new muscle weakness or pain, you need to call Dr. Johnson or me. We may need to lower the dose or switch to another medication. Other minor side effects include gas, constipation, stomach pain, and heartburn, but these tend to be mild and often go away. Fewer than 3 people out of 100 patients taking Lipitor have to stop taking it due to side effects.	Explain side effects of high frequency or clinical significance. Explain how to avoid/manage side effects. Explain drug interactions or medications to avoid.
I realize that you are not taking any other medications, but if you receive another prescription from Dr. Johnson or any other health care provider, we need to know about it.	

Rationale: Patients should know how to monitor themselves for critical side effects and what medications to avoid.

Conversation	Analysis
Dr. Perkins: Do you have any concerns about taking this medication?	Find out any barriers the patient perceives or hesitations he or she feels in beginning the therapy.
Ms. Burris: No. I know it is important to get my cholesterol down. It seems like it will be pretty simple to take this drug.	
Dr. Perkins: Just to be sure I haven't omitted any important information, please tell me how you are going to take the medication.	Ask for final verification of key information.

Case Study 8.6, cont.

Ms. Burris: I will probably take it at bedtime each night.	
Dr. Perkins: OK! What is the most significant side effect that you are going to watch for?	
Ms. Burris: That would be muscle pain or weakness.	
Dr. Perkins: That's right!	

Rationale: The key here is to (a) assess patient motivation to begin taking the drug and any barriers perceived to initiating therapy and (b) identify the essential information that patients must understand before they leave your pharmacy and verify that they do, in fact, understand.

Conversation	Analysis
Dr. Perkins: I have enjoyed talking to you about your medications. Here is the information leaflet that contains the material we just discussed plus additional information that I want you to read when you get home. Please let me know if you have questions about anything in there.	Provide an appropriate closing.
Ms. Burris: I will.	
Dr. Perkins: What other questions do you have for me now?	
Ms. Burris: None. I believe you covered everything pretty well.	
Dr. Perkins: Well, please call or stop by any time. I will call you in 2 weeks or so to make sure you are not having any problems. I will also check in after your visit with Dr. Johnson to hear how those cholesterol numbers are going.	Schedule follow-up to assess problems and monitor effectiveness of new therapies. Make yourself available in the future.
Thanks for coming in.	Thank the patient.

Rationale: For an appropriate closing: Encourage patients to contact you if they sense anything unusual or have any concern about their health status. Package the medication(s), give the patient the leaflet, and tell the patient to carefully read the leaflet and if anything causes them concern, to please call you, and you will be happy to discuss the problem. Conclude the transaction, and thank your patient.

REVIEW QUESTIONS

1. **What false assumptions do pharmacists often make that cloud otherwise clear communication?**
2. **What techniques can be used in patient education activities to help patients initiate medication therapy?**
3. **Describe three theoretical frameworks that can assist you in helping a patient change behavior.**
4. **Describe at least five techniques that help you motivate patients to change their behaviors in the direction of better health.**
5. **How can pharmacists help patients avoid reverting to old, unhealthy patterns of behavior after first implementing a change in a positive direction?**

REFERENCES

Agency for Healthcare Research and Quality. Evidence Report/Technology Assessment: Number 87. *Literacy and Health Outcomes*, 2005.

Bandura A. *Social Foundations of Thought and Action: A Social Cognitive Theory*. Englewood Cliffs, NJ: Prentice-Hall, 1986.

Butler JA, Roderick P, Mullee M, et al. Frequency and impact of nonadherence to immunosuppressants after renal transplantation: A systematic review. *Transplantation* 77:769–776, 2004.

Byrne M, Walsh J, Murphy AW. Secondary prevention of coronary heart disease: Patient beliefs and health-related behaviour. *Journal of Psychosomatic Research* 58:403–415, 2005.

Connor J, Rafter N, Rodgers A. Do fixed-dose combination pills or unit-of-use packaging improve adherence? A systematic review. *Bulletin World Health Organization* 82:935–939, 2004.

De Geest S, Moons P, Dobbels F, et al. Profiles of patients who experienced a late acute rejection due to nonadherence with immunosuppressive therapy. *Cardiovascular Nursing* 16:1–14, 2001.

DiMatteo MR. Social support and patient adherence to medical treatment: A meta-analysis. *Health Psychology* 23:207–218, 2004.

Doak CC, Doak LG, Root JH. The literacy problem. In *Teaching Patients with Low Literacy Skills* (2nd ed., pp. 1–9). Philadelphia, PA: J.B. Lippincott Co., 1996.

Gehi A, Haas D, Pipkin S, Whooley MA. Depression and medication adherence in outpatients with coronary heart disease: Findings from the Heart and Soul Study. *Archives of Internal Medicine* 165:2508–2513, 2005.

Godin G, Cote J, Naccache H, et al. Prediction of adherence to antiretroviral therapy: A one-year longitudinal study. *AIDS Care* 17:493–504, 2005.

Gonzalez JS, Penedo FJ, Antoni MH, et al. Social support, positive states of mind, and HIV treatment adherence in men and women living with HIV/AIDS. *Health Psychology* 23:413–418, 2004.

Hanchak NA, Patel MB, Berlin JA, Strom BL. Patient misunderstanding of dosing instructions. *Journal of General Internal Medicine* 11:325–328, 1996.

Institute of Medicine (IOM). *Crossing the Quality Chasm: A New Health System for the 21st Century*. Washington, DC:IOM, 2001.

Iskedjian M, Einarson TR, MacKeigan LD, et al. Relationship between daily dose frequency and adherence to antihypertensive pharmacotherapy: Evidence from a meta-analysis. *Clinical Therapeutics* 24:302–316, 2002.

Johnson MO, Catz SL, Remien RH, et al. Theory-guided, empirically supported avenues for intervention on HIV medication nonadherence: Findings from the Healthy Living Project. *AIDS Patient Care and STDS* 17:645–656, 2003.

Lewis MP, Colbert A, Erlen J, Meyers M. A qualitative study of persons who are 100% adherent to antiretroviral therapy. *AIDS Care* 18:140–148, 2006.

Maddigan SL, Majumdar SR, Johnson JA. Understanding the complex associations between patient-provider relationships, self-care behaviours, and health-related quality of life in type 2 diabetes: A structural equation modeling approach. *Quality of Life Research* 14:1489–1500, 2005.

Makoul G, Arntson P, Schofield T. Health promotion in primary care: Physician-patient communication and decision making about prescription medications. *Social Science and Medicine* 41: 1241–1254, 1995.

Marlatt GA, Parks GA, Witkiewitz K. *Clinical Guidelines for Implementing Relapse Prevention Therapy: A Guidebook Developed for the Behavioral Health Recovery Management Project*. Chicago: Illinois Department of Human Services, 2002.

Miller W, Rollnick S. *Motivational Interviewing: Preparing People for Change* (2nd ed.). New York, NY: Guilford Press, 2002.

Murphy DA, Marelich WD, Hoffman D, Steers WN. Predictors of antiretroviral adherence. *AIDS Care* 16:471–484, 2004.

Patel NC, Crismon ML, Miller AL, Johnsrud MT. Drug adherence: Effects of decreased visit frequency on adherence to clozapine therapy. *Pharmacotherapy* 25:1242–1247, 2005.

Phillips KD, Moneyham L, Murdaugh C, et al. Sleep disturbance and depression as barriers to adherence. *Clinical Nursing Research* 14:273–293, 2005.

Prochaska JO, DiClemente CC. Transtheoretical therapy: Toward a more integrative model of change. *Psychotherapy: Theory, Research and Practice* 19:276–288, 1982.

Prochaska JO, Norcross JC, DiClemente CC. *Changing for Good*. New York, NY: William Morrow and Company, Inc., 1994.

Rogers C. *Client-Centered Therapy*. New York, NY: Houghton Mifflin Company, 1951.

Rogers C. *On Becoming a Person*. New York, NY: Houghton Mifflin Company, 1961.

Royal Pharmaceutical Society of Great Britain and Merck Sharp & Dohme. *From Compliance to Concordance: Achieving Shared Goals in Medicine Taking*. London: Royal Pharmaceutical Society of Great Britain, 1997.

Sackett DL, Haynes RB. *Compliance with Therapeutic Regimens*. Baltimore, MD: The Johns Hopkins University Press, 1976.

Sherman J, Hutson A, Baumstein S, Hendeles L. Telephoning the patient's pharmacy to assess adherence with asthma medications by measuring refill rate for prescriptions. *Journal of Pediatrics* 136:532–536, 2000.

Smith DL. Compliance packaging: A powerful marketing tool. *Trends and Forecasts*. National Pharmaceutical Council, 1989; 2:3.

World Health Organization. Adherence to long-term therapies: Evidence for action. WHO, 2003, accessed September, 2010. http://www.who.int/chronic_conditions/adherencereport/en.

RECOMMENDED READINGS

Aljasem LI, Peyrot M, Wissow L, Rubin RR. The impact of barriers and self-efficacy on self-care behaviors in type 2 diabetes. *Diabetes Education* 27:393–404, 2001.

Ammassari A, Trotta MP, Murri R, et al. Correlates and predictors of adherence to highly active antiretroviral therapy: Overview of published literature. *Journal of Acquired Immune Deficiency Syndromes* 31(Suppl 3):S123–S127, 2002.

DiMatteo MR, Lepper HS, Croghan TW. Depression is a risk factor for noncompliance with medical treatment: Meta-analysis of the effects of anxiety and depression on patient adherence. *Archives of Internal Medicine* 160:2101–2107, 2000.

Marlatt GA, Gordon JR. *Relapse Prevention: Maintenance Strategies in the Treatment of Addictive Behaviors*. New York, NY: Guilford, 1985.

McKenney JM, et al. Impact of an electronic medication compliance aid on long-term blood pressure control. *Journal of Clinical Pharmacology* 32:277–283, 1992.

Perkins DO. Predictors of noncompliance in patients with schizophrenia. *Journal of Clinical Psychiatry* 63:1121–1128, 2002.

Svarstad BL. Patient-practitioner relationships and compliance with prescribed medical regimens. In Aiken, LH ed. *Application of Social Sciences to Clinical Medicine on Health Policy* (pp. 438–459). Rutgers, NJ: Rutgers University Press, 1986.

CHAPTER

9

Medication Safety and Communication Skills

Overview

As discussed in earlier chapters, effective communication skills are essential in ensuring that patients understand how to take their medications correctly. Moreover, recent experiences have illustrated that effective communication skills are also instrumental in ensuring patient safety in a variety of health care settings. This chapter explores the direct relationship between the quality of communication and the level of patient safety and focuses on how weak communication influences medication safety. It illustrates how many drug misadventures are caused by ineffective communication. For an example, see Case Study 9.1.

Introduction to Medication Safety Issues

What would happen if 200 Boeing 747 jetliners crashed each year? What would be the public's outcry? What would Congress do? Nearly 100,000 lives lost. Terrible and unimaginable! Yes, but according to an Institute of Medicine report, about the same number of Americans lose their lives to medication errors in hospitals each year (IOM, 2006). Although the accuracy of this estimate has been called into question, its relative importance cannot be ignored. Even if reality is just a tenth of that estimate, that is still a significant number of preventable deaths due to error. Other estimates indicate that more than 1.5 million Americans (about the population of the state of Idaho) will experience some type of medication error each

CASE STUDY 9.1

Brenda Anderson, a 78-year-old white female, visited her physician for a refill of her "blood thinner" (Coumadin 5.0 mg). Based on her recent lab work, Brenda's physician told her to take one-half a tablet daily for 4 days and then 1 tablet daily thereafter. Her physician wrote a prescription for:

Coumadin 5.0 mg. SIG: 2½ mg q.d. × 4 d; 1 tab q.d. #30.

John Coleman, the pharmacist who filled Brenda's prescription, typed 2½ tablets daily for 4 days and then one tablet daily on the prescription label. Unfortunately, John was too busy to speak with Brenda when she picked up her prescription. While at home, Brenda forgot what her physician said (she was nervous, as she always is at the doctor's office) and followed John's instructions. Thus, she took 2½ tablets (five times the amount that was intended!). Going into her 4th day of this treatment, Brenda died of massive hemorrhaging. This situation is based on an actual case experience.

year. In addition, the IOM report states that medication errors have a significant economic impact as well. The annual cost of drug-related morbidity and mortality in the United States has been estimated to be more than $140 billion.

It is beyond the scope of this chapter to discuss the entire corpus of medication error literature or to probe into the many possible causes and potential solutions regarding such errors. The suggested readings at the end of this chapter will provide this type of analysis for the reader. This chapter focuses on the role of inappropriate counseling and communication in causing medication errors, and the role that effective communication skills have in preventing medication errors.

Health care providers have always been concerned with safety, but research reveals that preventable medication errors still occur at unacceptable rates (Cohen, 1999; Friedman et al., 2009). What do we mean by "medication error"? According to the National Coordinating Council for Medication Error Reporting and Prevention (NCCMERP), the definition of medication error is "… any preventable event that may cause or lead to inappropriate medication use or patient harm while the medication is in the control of the health care provider, patient, or consumer" (NCCMERP, 2005).

Medication errors not only cause physical harm to patients, but also undermine patient confidence in the health care system. Patients may perceive medications in a different light and may not trust information provided by health care providers. These perceptions may directly affect patient adherence with prescribed therapy or may stimulate the use of alternative therapies. Medication errors also cause tension between health care providers. Fingerpointing may occur, and perceptions of professional competence may be altered. When situations are not handled appropriately, trust evaporates and future interactions do not evolve in a positive way.

It is easy to say that medication errors are either "system" problems or "people" problems. All we need to do is to fix the system or train people better to decrease errors. While developing better health care delivery systems and more effective training programs will enhance patient safety, preventing medication errors is a complex process and multiple approaches are needed to remedy harmful situations.

Take Mrs. Anderson's situation in Case Study 9.1 as an example—was this death related to a system failure or a pharmacist's personal error? John, the pharmacist who filled the prescription, obviously misinterpreted the directions (2½ tablets rather than 2½ mg), so it is easy to just blame him. However, although John bears some responsibility for this error, he may not be entirely culpable. Possibly the physician's handwriting was not clear, thus "mg" might have looked like "tab." The physician could have written the prescription more clearly. He wrote the directions in an unorthodox way (2½ mg rather than 2.5 mg). Thus, John's eyes saw the 2½ and inferred that it related to how many tablets should be given. Physicians typically use fractions when indicating how many tablets. Being a refill prescription, John might have rationalized that he did not need to talk to Mrs. Anderson because she had been taking this drug for a long time and knew how to take it. In addition, system errors may have led to John's misinterpretation. Possibly he was under stress and was working too fast (his assistant called in sick and thus he was short of staff). Possibly his ability to see clearly was hindered by inadequate lighting in the pharmacy. Patient issues also might have influenced the tragic outcome. Possibly Mrs. Anderson did not remember what her physician told her about how the medication was to be taken. If she had remembered, she would have detected the error as soon as she read the prescription label, and John could have remedied the situation.

Let's analyze how elements of the communication model impacted this situation. First of all, the physician could have *transmitted* his message more clearly by writing down his instructions for Mrs. Anderson during her office visit, but he chose to rely on her memory instead. The physician could have *transmitted* the prescription via an electronic physician order system to the pharmacy, thus eliminating any doubt about his intentions. John could have *asked for clarification* of the physician's message by calling the physician about the instructions once he noticed that the dose was written in an unorthodox manner (2½ vs. 2.5). John could have carved out time to counsel Mrs. Anderson and *ask* her how she was supposed to take the medication. This was especially important since the new directions were different from her previous prescriptions (1 tablet daily as recorded in her profile). In addition, John could have *asked for feedback* from Mrs. Anderson by checking to see whether she *understood* that she had to change regimens in just a few days. This discussion may have caused Mrs. Anderson to remember her physician's original instructions. John could have encouraged Mrs. Anderson to *contact* him if she had any questions and to always *question* anything that did not look right.

Types of Errors: Possible Causes and Potential Solutions

As highlighted by the above example, medication errors typically involve complex relationships between systems, people, and communication processes. This section discusses the most common types of medication errors involving the communication process directly or indirectly.

COMMUNICATION WITH HEALTH CARE PROVIDERS

Possible Issues

As in the Brenda Anderson situation in Case Study 9.1, many errors occur in the process of physicians communicating instructions to pharmacists and in the pharmacist's ability to interpret these instructions (Dayton and Henriksen, 2007). Regardless of setting (institutional or community practice), prescribers might not convey their messages clearly, and pharmacists might not have an opportunity to provide feedback regarding their interpretation and understanding of these messages. Within institutional environments, similar issues involve pharmacist communication with nurses, physical therapists, dietitians, and other health care providers. Thousands of messages (instructions, drug information, patient information, etc.) are sent each day; many times these are not communicated clearly or interpreted correctly. This is true for both written and verbal communication. Common issues involving verbal communication include:

- Distractions and noise that interfere with clear transmission and receipt of the message
- Heavy accents and language differences
- Use of terminology that other health care providers do not understand
- Speaking too rapidly for the listener to clearly comprehend
- Medications that sound alike when spoken (Zantac vs. Zyrtec)
- Numbers that sound alike (15 vs. 50; 19 vs. 90)

Although written communication is often preferred over verbal communication to minimize errors, there are several issues that inhibit effective written communication as well. Examples of written communication issues include:

- Poor handwriting
- Medication names that look alike when written out (Celexa vs. Celebrex or Bisoprolol 10 mg and Buspirone 10 mg)
- Misplaced zeroes and decimal points in dosing instructions (.5 vs. 0.5; 1.0 vs. 10)
- Unclear abbreviations within patient care instructions

The real-life situation described in Case Study 9.2 illustrates the potential problems with written communication within hospitals.

CASE STUDY 9.2

In a large teaching hospital, a physician wrote an order for morphine PO, which was transcribed by the nurse as morphine IV since intravenous medications were used more than oral meds in her unit. The patient received three times the desired dose, went into respirator depression, and eventually died. Following this situation, physicians in this hospital who are found using illegible handwriting are now fined and required to take handwriting courses.

Potential Strategies

The following may serve to minimize the issues described above. In general, you should be able to contact colleagues at any time to clarify issues regarding patient therapy. You should also review the possible barriers discussed in previous chapters (perceptual, environmental, etc.) that may be inhibiting communication with health care providers. For example

- Work load issues may prevent you from contacting physicians or nurses.
- Elements within the work environment may promote distractions and prevent you from concentrating on your work.
- The layout of the work area may not be appropriate.
- The lighting within the pharmacy area may not be adequate.
- Communication networks (phone, e-mail, text-messaging, etc.) may not provide easy access to professionals so that you can provide feedback.
- Indirect communication (i.e., you talk to a nurse who talks with the physician rather than you talking directly with the physician).

Resolving these general issues may minimize medication errors and their negative outcomes. During the dispensing process, the work flow should include numerous opportunities to check the contents and labels of prescriptions. Several pharmacies use bar coding (see Figure 9-1) as a means to check the accuracy of the dispensing process. Many pharmacists advocate using "Tall Man Lettering" when writing drug names that are similar to other agents (e.g., using glipiZIDE and glyBURIDE rather than glipizide and glyburide within the prescription order and on the prescription label). Another example would be to use "chlorproPAMIDE" and "chlorproMAZINE" to differentiate between these two agents that look very similar but have very different uses. To minimize errors when taking verbal orders over the phone, you should repeat all components of a verbal order and place a checkmark on the prescription for each component as you read it back to the prescriber.

In institutional settings, such as long-term care facilities, hospitals, or ambulatory care centers, communication between pharmacy and nursing staffs must be clear to assure safe administration of the medication (Golz and Fitchett, 1999). For example, is the medication labeled clearly? Are doses appropriate? Are the instructions for delivery method (IM, IV) and administration times clearly articulated? Within these institutions, staff members need to be trained in the proper communication processes and educated about the potential causes of medication errors. You must work closely with these professionals to ensure accurate interpretation of orders and administration of medications. It is also critical to have access to the most up-to-date drug information references for health care providers, preferably in an electronic format, so that the most current information is used.

COMMUNICATION WITH PATIENTS

Possible Issues

As revealed in Mrs. Anderson's situation in Case Study 9.1 and in other cases involving medication errors, multiple opportunities exist for communication

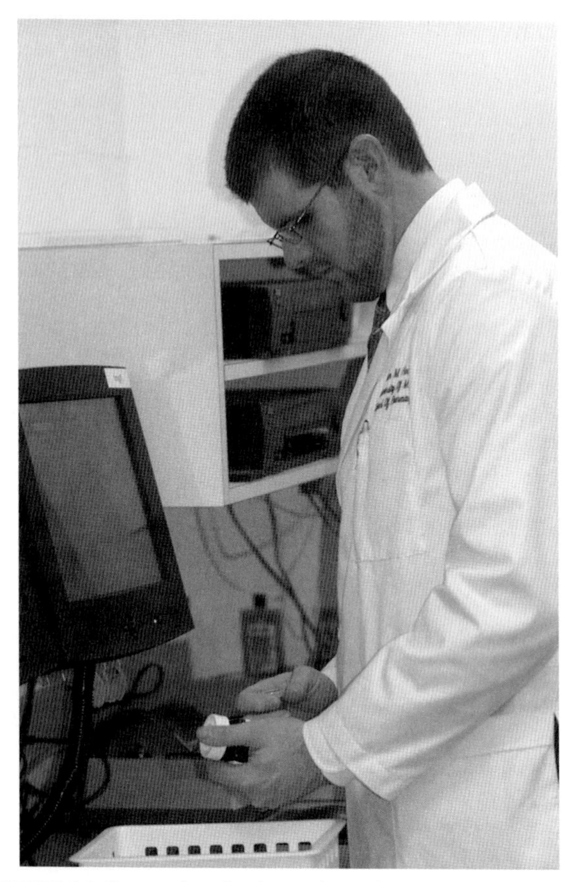

FIGURE 9-1. Pharmacist using bar-code reader to minimize errors.

failure between pharmacists and patients. Common issues involving verbal communication include:

- Inability of patients to understand pharmacists (accent, medical terminology, language and cultural differences, etc.)
- Hearing and vision impairments
- Environmental barriers (noisy pharmacy, no access to pharmacist)

Common issues involving written communication with patients include:

- Patient's inability to read or comprehend material
- Lack of effective patient education material
- Inability to read label (sight impairments)

Other pharmacist–patient communication issues leading to medication errors include:

- Pharmacist's failure to make sure the correct patient receives the right medication (is the Mary Jones picking up a prescription the right Mary Jones?)
- Patient's reluctance to question and lack of encouragement to clarify verbal and written information with pharmacists

Potential Strategies

Many situations involve patient interaction within the pharmacy, while others occur after the patient leaves the pharmacy. Fortunately, many errors are discovered during the pharmacist–patient counseling interaction and are corrected before patients leave the pharmacy (Ukens, 1997). For this to occur, however, patients need to be actively involved with their drug therapy. Their participation could identify potential errors. Patients and their caregivers should realize they have a stake in preventing errors. Patients should feel free to question situations that do not appear right and mention them to you.

When giving information to patients, you should allow patients the opportunity to repeat back key information in order to detect possible errors and misunderstandings. Counseling should be used to verify the accuracy of dispensing and to assess patient understanding of proper medication use. When giving verbal instructions, difficult drug names should be spelled out for patients. Written patient education leaflets should be given for future reference. As stated in other sections of the book, patient education material must be targeted at an appropriate reading level. It is estimated that more than 90 million Americans have limited health literacy skills (Nielsen-Bohlman et al., 2004). You should use the Internet and smart phone technologies as effective mechanisms to communicate with patients. You should keep notes in your patient database about unique patient characteristics (hearing, speech, or vision impairments). You should also document past issues involving errors or nonadherence to therapy within the patient's profile.

You should encourage your patients to keep a list of all their medications and instructions along with critical health information, such as drug allergies. Patients should refer to their lists every time they visit their physicians or pharmacists; being proactive will minimize patient risk. You should offer advice on how patients can minimize their exposure to medication errors. Patients need to know what the medication is used for, how to take it, what to expect, and other essential information. If their therapy changes from one visit to the next, patients should feel comfortable bringing it to your attention. Unfortunately, this does not occur all the time. As discussed in other chapters, you might use the "show and tell" technique of showing the medication to the patient and asking the patient what the medication is used for and how they are taking it. This approach can alert both the patient and you to possible issues before the patient leaves the pharmacy. In fact, one study found that 89% of the errors that had made it through the medication processing steps and the final pharmacist check were caught at the point of patient counseling when pharmacists showed the medication to patients and verified its indication of use with them (Kuyper, 1993). As an example, see Case Study 9.3.

CASE STUDY 9.3

A patient enters Morgan's Pharmacy and presents a prescription for:
Indocin 25 mg SIG: 1 cap bid prn #20
After filling the prescription, the pharmacist counsels the patient as follows.

Pharmacist: What exactly are you taking Indocin for?

Patient: I'm taking it for diarrhea.

Pharmacist: Diarrhea, huh? Did your doctor and you discuss the need for a pain medication?

Patient: No, just diarrhea. I feel fine otherwise.

Pharmacist: Let me double-check something here; I will be right back.

The pharmacist then calls the prescribing physician to inform him about the patient's statement. The physician says: "Oh my goodness, I meant to prescribe Imodium, I must have been thinking about another patient I just saw in clinic with back pain. Thanks for calling about this one. Please change the prescription to Imodium 2 mg." This situation is based on an actual experience.

In Case Study 9.3, the pharmacist was able to identify a prescribing error by simply asking the patient an open-ended question. Using this approach, she was able to determine the patient's perception about what the medication was used for. She also asked if there might be a pain issue involved (possibly Indocin was prescribed for a pain-related issue and the actual treatment for the diarrhea was not clear to the patient; possibly the physician forgot to write a prescription, or possibly the patient was to treat the diarrhea in some other manner). Once the patient indicated that diarrhea was the only health issue, the pharmacist realized that something was not right and excused herself before making any other statements to the patient. She then called the physician to clarify things and thus resolved the error.

General Strategies to Enhance Patient Safety

While the previous section addressed specific causes and strategies for dealing with errors, broader strategies exist that need to be considered to enhance overall medication safety. Using these general approaches, you can minimize medication errors in your practice setting.

REPORTING ERRORS

You should establish a culture within your practice environment that recognizes that errors do occur and should be reported so the system can be improved. It is important to establish a nonpunitive approach to dealing with errors to minimize feelings of embarrassment, fear, or lack of professionalism that many people feel once an error is discovered. Most people are reluctant to report an error, or they try to work around the error without letting others know about it. In addition, peers are reluctant to report errors made by their colleagues. It is important to realize that most errors are caught by others. We rarely catch our own errors. So we must rely on others to find and report errors using the various levels of quality control.

To be most effective, reporting mechanisms should not be punitive, but should be instructive. People should not lose their jobs or be penalized (except in cases of dereliction of duty or criminal activity) when errors occur. The aviation and automobile industries found out the hard way that penalizing employees actually increased potential errors by decreasing the number of reported errors and near misses and by eliminating any opportunity to remedy structural or procedural deficiencies. Many errors are related to system issues rather than people issues. Thus, people must feel comfortable identifying, documenting, and reporting errors in a constructive environment. The organization's philosophy and culture should be nonpunitive, which is difficult at times. A delicate balance exists between holding personnel to a high level of quality and professionalism and at the same time recognizing that some errors will occur and that employees are not to be punished when errors are reported.

You should develop protocols to use when errors occur and to develop appropriate methods to report errors. Furthermore, staff may have different perceptions of what an error actually is. Thus, examples of possible errors must be included in training so individuals understand what needs to be monitored and reported. Unfortunately, many errors are not detected, but for those that are found, they should be documented and reported. Reporting systems must be user-friendly, quick, and easy to use. Documenting errors (in a dedicated logbook or on the back of the prescription) provides a clear paper trail for further analysis. This documentation may also be helpful in future interactions with specific patients or prescribers. Not reporting errors prevents the creation of a clear picture of possible issues. People sometimes rationalize that it was a one-time slip-up when in actuality it might be occurring all the time. Without proper documentation and reporting, individual pharmacists, their managers, and the entire department are not aware of specific issues that need to be addressed. Thus, departments are destined to continue to repeat the same error. It is important to report "near misses" as well, including how the error was prevented and how it might not have been prevented under other circumstances. Periodic studies of past errors need to be implemented in order to establish possible trends leading to eventual plans to correct them. Continuous training is essential to minimize future errors.

Several national reporting efforts have been established to track errors and their potential causes. The MedMARX program (see Box 9.1 for contact information) is an anonymous reporting system used by hospitals and health care organizations to share information regarding patient safety and medication errors. The United States Pharmacopeia (USP) Medication Errors Reporting Program

Box 9.1 Relevant Web Sites

- Institute for Safe Medication Practices: www.ismp.org
- National Patient Safety Foundation: www.npsf.org
- National Coordinating Council on Medication Error Reporting and Prevention: www.nccmerp.org
- AHCPR-Medical Errors & Patient Safety Subdirectory Page: www.ahcpr.gov/qual/errors.htm
- Quality Interagency Coordination (QuIC) Task Force: www.quic.gov
- USP Medication Errors Reporting Program: www.usp.org and 1–800–23ERROR
- MEDMARX: www.usp.org/ and 1–877-MEDMARX
- AHRQ brochure "20 Tips to Prevent Medical Errors": www.ahrq.gov

(see Box 9.1) is a confidential and anonymous reporting system for health care professionals who encounter actual or potential medication errors. According to the USP program, "By reporting errors, pharmacists, nurses, physicians, and other healthcare practitioners contribute to improved patient safety and to the development of valuable educational services for the prevention of future errors." The USP forwards all information to the FDA as a partner in the FDA's MedWatch program so that information can be entered into this important database. The Institute for Safe Medication Practices also assists USP in the development and implementation of the Medication Errors Reporting Program. You should be encouraged to report errors to these national systems to help identify medication safety issues.

ORGANIZED STRATEGIES TO MINIMIZE ERRORS

Several strategies have been used by safety experts to identify the causes of errors within a variety of work environments. Many of these approaches can be adapted to pharmacy practice settings, such as Failure Mode and Effects Analysis (FMEA) and Root Cause Analysis (RCA) (Cohen, 1999). FMEA attempts to identify sources of potential failure within a specific system and the consequences of such failures. It can be used to evaluate previous failures or to prevent future failures. The goal of this risk management tool is to reduce the frequency of failures and minimize their consequences. RCA focuses on specific root causes of errors and not on the actual errors themselves; it attempts to identify the specific reasons for the error by asking a series of probing "why" questions to eventually find the root cause. Many times, RCA discovers multiple causes of the error, resulting in numerous opportunities for change. Pharmacists in institutional practice settings may be more familiar with these approaches than their community practice colleagues. However, many experts urge that these strategies can be used in a variety of pharmacy practice settings and can be used to evaluate communication and patient counseling issues.

General risk management systems can also be used to minimize procedural and personnel issues. Risk management does not necessarily mean risk elimination; errors will still occur, but hopefully in fewer numbers, with less severity, and before they harm patients. Effective risk management systems decrease the incidence of preventable errors and lessen the consequences of errors that cannot be prevented (Abood, 2005). Quality assurance programs will assist in improving risk management. You should become familiar with the risk management and quality assurance programs within your practice setting. You also are encouraged to work with risk managers and other professionals in this area to implement strategies to minimize errors. The key is to develop and implement standards and best practices and to implement quality improvement systems in order to decrease the potential for error.

When Errors Occur

What do you do when an error occurs? How do you handle the embarrassing situation of telling someone that you made an error? What do you do when an injury or death has occurred (as in Brenda Anderson's situation in Case Study 9.1)? Difficult questions to face, but as revealed in this section, effective communication skills can help you respond appropriately in these situations. Put another way, weak communication skills can certainly make situations worse. Readers should be aware that legal counsel must be consulted if there is a chance of litigation surrounding the event. Thus, readers are encouraged to consult material written from the legal perspective (Abood, 2005). This chapter focuses only on the communication skills related to the discovery and disclosure of medication errors.

INITIAL DISCOVERY

When an error occurs, you must make sure the patient is not harmed or does not continue to be at risk. Thus, timely intervention is critical to an effective resolution. The first general response to finding an error might be:

- **Avoidance:** "I didn't make the error; it is not my responsibility to get involved." "My boss should deal with it."
- **Blaming someone or something else:** "The physician's poor handwriting was the problem." "The computer system went down."
- **Rationalizing that the error was not important:** "It is no big deal that I gave Terramycin tablets rather than capsules."
- **Rationalizing that the patient will call the pharmacy if there is a problem.**

INITIAL CONTACT WITH PATIENT

The first few moments of contact with patients are critical in determining how the situation will eventually be resolved. You want to appear to be in control of the situation (that you are working to resolve the situation), but at the same time allow the patient to state his or her feelings. If the patient is in the pharmacy, go with him or her to a quiet area where other people cannot overhear. When patients learn about a particular error, they typically want to hear a brief description of exactly what happened and the short-term consequences of the error ("This dose might increase your chances of having diarrhea"). They also want to be reassured that you are trying to resolve the situation immediately. Patients need to perceive that you are genuinely concerned about the error and are taking immediate steps to deal with it. If they perceive that you are not too concerned, they may be more prone to litigation.

During the initial contact, you should make a simple, but clear statement that you are extremely sorry for the error. You should not place the blame on technology ("The computer didn't catch the error"), other people ("The evening pharmacist made the error"), or the fact that you were too busy. If you found the error, you need to take the responsibility for trying to resolve it. If your assistant made the error, you, as the pharmacist in charge, should not transfer blame to him or her since the error occurred under your watch. Also, you should not suggest that the patient might have contributed to the problem: "You should have called before you took a dose of medication you thought was wrong." Do not minimize the importance of the error: "Luckily, no harm was done. Taking the 1 mg strength of Xanax instead of the 2 mg wouldn't have hurt you." Patients are initially more concerned about the fact that an error has occurred regardless of its potential harm.

Some errors can be remedied relatively easily ("Please bring the prescription into the pharmacy and we will give you the new prescription" or "Our staff will be bringing the new prescription out to your home later today"), while others might be more complex and may take time to resolve ("I need to discuss this situation with your physician before making a decision about what needs to be done"). In situations that may take additional time, you need to convey that fact to the patient so he or she feels that you are still concerned and are working toward a resolution and did not just forget about it.

Finally, you should thank the patient for bringing the error to your attention: "Thank you for checking your medicine and telling us immediately that you had a concern." Even when patients think an error has occurred but one has not (e.g., a different-looking generic was dispensed), you should thank them for being vigilant and reporting the possible error. Your communication should encourage patients to always bring a concern about a medication to your attention before beginning to take the medication.

FURTHER CONTACT

Once the patient has a clear idea that an error has occurred and how it is being resolved, you may want to provide additional insights into why it occurred. Some patients might want to know how it occurred and what steps you are going to implement to prevent future occurrences. It is best to monitor the patient's interest before launching into a detailed explanation. Some patients might not care since they are only focusing on their own situation. To some patients, a lengthy explanation may seem like you are making excuses. You should be honest and upfront with the patient about the long-term consequences of the error. They may be interested to learn how they will be compensated for their inconvenience or injury. You should make sure that you do not rush through the experience and allow patients time to ask questions and express their feelings. On the other hand, you do not want to prolong the process either or keep repeating the same phrases. You should encourage patient expressions about what they are thinking and feeling about the situation. This feedback will help you determine whether you need to conclude the interaction or continue to address the patient's remaining concerns.

A sincere closing statement, such as "This rarely happens, but it happened with your prescription and I want to resolve it," may put the error in perspective. Patients need to hear that you found an error, you feel terrible about it, it does not happen that often, but it did happen to them, and you are going to try to resolve it. You should also contact them at a later time to determine whether they have additional questions and update them with relevant information. Finally, you should write everything down for future reference (especially if litigation occurs). Documentation is also helpful for your quality assurance program and for the national reporting systems as well.

CONTACTING OTHER HEALTH CARE PROVIDERS

You should alert physicians or other health care providers if they were involved with the original error (poor handwriting, wrong drug prescribed, prescribing two medications that interact with each other, etc.) or if the patient requires treatment due to damage caused by the error. Once again, you may be tempted to avoid contacting others since you may be embarrassed or concerned that your professional competence may be called into question. However, if you do not report it and they find out through the patient or some other means, then you will suffer additional consequences. Your colleagues will be observing how you handle the error. If they perceive that you are handling it appropriately, they will be inclined to forgive the error and move on. However, if not, they may not trust your veracity or professional competence in the future. Finally, revealing errors to other providers is helpful for their quality assurance efforts as well. They need to know how they may have personally contributed to the error and how communication and/or other elements of the "system" need to be improved to minimize future errors.

Summary

Medication errors typically involve complex relationships between systems, people, and communication processes. They typically involve issues within and outside the control of patients, pharmacists, and other care providers. Patients are certainly concerned about medication errors. In fact, a recent study found that 69% of all hospitalized patients were concerned about "being given the wrong medicine" while staying in the hospital (American Society of Health-System Pharmacists, 2002). As outlined above, pharmacists and their staffs need to be aware of the possible communication issues that may lead to medication errors. They should reflect on errors that are identified within their practice setting and eventually use this information to improve the quality of care. The key is to develop and implement standards of practice that minimize errors and to implement quality improvement systems in order to decrease the potential for error.

REVIEW QUESTIONS

1. **What is the definition of a medication error?**
2. **What are the various national medication error reporting programs?**
3. **Name two strategies for risk reduction.**
4. **What elements of the communication model are most critical to the communication process surrounding medication errors?**

REFERENCES

Abood, R. *Pharmacy Practice and the Law* (4th ed.). Sudbury, MA: Jones and Bartlett Publishers, 2005.

American Society of Health-System Pharmacists 2002 Omnibus Survey. 2002. *Top patient concerns.* Retrieved August 20, 2006 from http://www.ashp.org/ pr/SurveyReport.pdf.

Cohen MR. *Medication Errors: Causes, Prevention and Risk Management.* Sudbury MA: Jones & Bartlett, 1999.

Dayton E, Henriksen K. The role of communication failures in medical errors. *Joint Commission Journal on Quality and Patient Safety* 33(1):34–47, 2007.

Friedman B, Encinosa W, Jiang H, et al., The effects of adverse safety events in the hospital on risks of death and readmission. *Medical Care* 47(5):583–590, 2009.

Golz G, Fitchett L. Nurses' perspective on a serious adverse drug event. *American Journal of Hospital Pharmacy* 56:904–907, 1999.

Institute of Medicine. *Preventing Medication Errors: Quality Chasm Series.* Washington, DC: National Academy Press, 2006.

Kuyper AR. Patient counseling detects prescription errors. *Hospital Pharmacy* 28:1180–1182, 1993.

NCCMERP: National Coordinating Council on Medication Error Reporting and Prevention. 2005. Retrieved August 20, 2006, from http://www.nccmerp.org.

Nielsen-Bohlman L, Panzer AM, Kindig DA (eds.). *Health Literacy: A Prescription to End Confusion.* Washington, DC: National Academy Press, 2004.

Ukens C. Deadly dispensing: An exclusive survey of Rx errors by pharmacists. *Drug Topics* 141:100–111, 1997.

RECOMMENDED READINGS

American Society of Health-system Pharmacists. *Best Practices for Health-System Pharmacy* (pp. 149–159). Bethesda, MD: ASHP, 2004.

Brushwood DB. *The Power of Words: Responding Appropriately to a Patient's Concerns about Quality*. Washington, DC: Institute for the Advancement of Community Pharmacy, 2001.

Grasha AF. Pharmacy workload: The causes and confusion behind dispensing errors. *Canadian Pharmaceutical Journal* 134:26–35, 2001.

Institute of Medicine. *To Err is Human: Building a Safer Health System*. Washington, DC: National Academy Press,2000.

Johnson JA, Bootman JL. Drug-related morbidity and mortality: A cost-of-illness model. *Archives of Internal Medicine* 155:1949–1956, 1995.

Johnson JA, Bootman JL. Drug-related morbidity and mortality and the economic impact of pharmaceutical care. *American Journal of Hospital Pharmacy* 54:554–558, 1997.

Lambert BL. Predicting look-alike and sound-alike medication errors. *American Journal of Hospital Pharmacy* 54:1161–1171, 1997.

Manasse HR. Medication use in an imperfect world: Drug misadventuring as an issue of public policy. *American Journal of Hospital Pharmacy* Part 1: 46:436–439; Part 2: 46:1141–1152, 1989.

Morrison PE, Helneke J. Why do health care practitioners resist quality management? *Quality Progress* 25:51–55, 1992.

Reason J. *Human Error*. Cambridge: Cambridge University Press, 1990.

CHAPTER

10

Strategies to Meet Specific Needs

Overview

Applying interpersonal communication skills in pharmacy practice is not always easy. It can become especially difficult in situations where patients bring special communication needs. These situations require special sensitivities and unique strategies to ensure that effective communication between pharmacist and patient takes place. This chapter addresses several interpersonal communication skills necessary to deal with the following:

- Older adults
- Persons with hearing, sight, or speech impairments
- Patients with disabilities
- Terminally ill patients
- Patients with sexually communicated infections, such as HIV/AIDS
- Patients with mental health problems
- Patients with limited health literacy

- Patients from different cultural backgrounds
- Persons who serve as caregivers

This chapter provides practical means of recognizing those individuals with unique communication needs and offers strategies that can be used to overcome challenges to interpersonal communication effectiveness.

Introduction

Communication in pharmacy practice is frequently hindered by specific challenges presented by unique groups of patients who present with special communication needs. This chapter discusses specific communication barriers involving a variety of situations. Different strategies are also outlined to assist you in identifying and dealing with these special communication needs. It is important to remember that one approach might work with one patient, but not others, so you need to have a variety of strategies in mind as you approach these situations.

Before discussing the unique communication challenges of these patients, one caveat that applies to most situations must be offered: If you sense that a person has a unique problem, you should check your perception of that problem (see Chapter 3 about how we act based on our perceptions of the patient). An example is how we often treat older adults. While some older patients may appear to be frail, they may not be forgetful or hard of hearing. However, we make certain assumptions based on our perceptions of the elderly as a group of patients. Thus, we may start raising our voice or talking slower. The key is to assess how they are responding to your educational efforts. You should watch for nonverbal clues to see whether they are leaning toward you or whether they have a confused look. Asking open-ended questions can also provide feedback about the patient's ability to communicate. Not checking initial impressions could lead to potentially embarrassing situations for both patients and you. You should try to avoid stereotyping individuals and make sure to check your perceptions.

Older Adults

The number of older adults in our society is increasing, and they consume a disproportionate amount of prescription and nonprescription medications when compared with other age groups. Men and women over the age of 65 present special opportunities for pharmacists because they account for about 30% of all prescription medication taken in the United States and about 40% of all over-the-counter medication. Two out of three persons in this age group take at least one medication daily. Thus, this growing segment of the population is in need of your patient counseling services. Unfortunately, the aging process sometimes affects certain elements of communication, which can lead to more medication-related problems. These potential communication problems are discussed below.

LEARNING

In certain individuals, the aging process affects the learning process, but not the ability to learn. Some older adults learn at a slower rate than younger persons. They have the ability to learn, but they process information at a different rate. Thus, the rate of speech and the amount of information presented at one time must meet the individual's ability to comprehend the material. In addition, short-term memory, recall, and attention span may be diminished in some elderly patients. The ability to process new and innovative solutions to problems might also be slower in some older adults. Thus, attempts to change behaviors should be structured gradually and should build on past experiences. A good approach with some older adults is to set reasonable short-term goals, approach long-term goals in stages, and break down learning tasks into smaller components. Another important step is to encourage feedback from patients as to whether they received your intended message by asking them to summarize instructions and other information and by watching their nonverbal responses. When given the opportunity to learn at their own speed, most elderly people can learn as well as younger adults.

DIFFERENCES IN PERSPECTIVES

Potential communication barriers between you and older patients may be attributable to the generation gap. Some older adults may perceive things differently from those in different age groups since people typically adhere to values learned and accepted in their younger years. Thus, some older adults may have different beliefs and perceptions about health care in general and about drugs and pharmacists specifically. Some behaviors, such as hoarding and sharing medication, may seem inappropriate to you, but such actions may make sense to someone who grew up during the Depression or World War II. You should be aware of situations in which you may be reacting to older patients' different values and belief systems rather than to the patients themselves.

The image of the pharmacist and the pharmacy profession is also important. Older patients may expect a well-groomed, clean-shaven, professional-looking practitioner to serve them. If you do not meet these expectations, they may be somewhat reluctant to interact with you initially. Their perception of authority may also influence how they interact with you. Some older adults grew up respecting the social authority given to physicians and pharmacists and prefer a more directed approach to receiving health care. Thus, they may be receptive to being told what to do. On the other hand, many patients want to be more independent and may feel the need to assert themselves. They may be somewhat more demanding, want additional information, or want more input into the medication decision-making process. Thus, it is important to assess which approach seems to work for each patient.

SENSE OF LOSS

Some older adults may be experiencing a significant amount of loss compared with people of other age groups. For example, their friends may be dying at an increased rate, they may have retired from their jobs, or they may have had to slow down or cease certain activities due to the aging process. All these situations involve loss and subsequent grieving. Thus, their reaction to certain medical situations, such as ignoring your directions or complaining about the price of their medications, may be responses to fear of their diseases, of becoming even less active, or of dying. They may deny the situation or become angry at you or other health care providers. They may also turn to self-diagnosis and self-treatment or to the use of other people's medications.

VISUAL IMPAIRMENTS

If you work with elderly patients, you need to realize that the aging process may affect the visual process. Be prepared to offer alternative forms of patient counseling to deal with these impairments. Written messages for persons with visual deficiencies should be in large print and on pastel-colored paper rather than on white paper. Many times visual acuity is not as sharp, and sensitivity to color is decreased. In some older patients, more light is needed to stimulate the receptors in the eye. Thus, when using written information, make sure you have enough light.

HEARING LOSS

The aging process may also affect hearing. Auditory loss in various degrees of severity is seen in more than 50% of all older adults. The hearing loss associated with the aging process is called presbycusis. Unfortunately, this condition may lead individuals to withdraw socially and psychologically or, in extreme cases, may lead others to label them as senile or forgetful. Many older adults describe their hearing impairment as being able to hear what others are saying, but not being able to understand what is being said. They can hear words, but they cannot put them together clearly. Other types of hearing loss seen in some older adults are related to diminished response to high-frequency sounds. In some older adults, sensitivity to sound is decreased, and the volume must be increased to stimulate the receptors.

Three general types of physical hearing impairment (conductive, sensorineural, and central) can occur singly or in combination with one another. Conductive hearing impairment results when something blocks the conduction of sound into the ear's sensory nerve centers. Sensorineural impairment occurs when the problem is situated in the sensory center of the inner ear. Central hearing impairment occurs when the nerve centers within the brain are affected. A hearing aid is helpful for people with conductive hearing problems, less effective for those with sensorineural impairment, and ineffective for those with central loss. Because the hearing aid only makes the sound louder, it is not as helpful in patients who cannot distinguish sounds easily and may actually make some situations worse. Hearing deficiencies can also be caused by a variety of factors, including birth defects, injuries, and chronic exposure to loud noises.

Response to high-frequency sounds is usually diminished before the response to lower-frequency sounds. Thus, using a lower tone of voice may help some older adults. In some older persons, sensitivity to sound is decreased, and increased volume can assist in hearing. It is also important to slow your rate of speech somewhat so the person can differentiate the words. Remember not to shout when speaking, since shouting may offend some people. Talking in a somewhat higher volume may be necessary, but more likely a slower rate of speech will help most individuals. Finally, be aware of environmental barriers, such as loud background noises or dimly lit counseling areas, which make communication difficult for the hearing-impaired.

Many individuals with hearing deficiencies, including some older adults, rely on speech-reading (watching the lips, facial expressions, and gestures) to enhance their communication ability. Speech-reading is more than just lip-reading. It involves receiving visual cues from facial expressions, body postures, and gestures as well as lip movements. Research has shown that everyone develops some speech-reading skill and that the hearing-impaired typically develop that skill much further. Development of this skill is hindered if sight is impaired as well, as in some older adults. For speech-reading to be most effective, you should position patients directly in front of you and have a light shining on your lips and face when communicating.

To improve communication with hearing-impaired patients, try to position yourself about 3 to 6 feet away; never speak directly into the patient's ear because this may distort the message. Wait until the patient can see you before speaking; position yourself on the side of the patient's strongest ear; if necessary, touch the patient on the arm. If your message does not appear to be getting through, you should not keep repeating the same statement, but rephrase it into shorter, simpler sentences. Many pharmacists and their staffs have learned sign language to assist hearing-impaired patients.

SPEECH

In addition to decreased sight and hearing capacity, some elderly might have slight or significant speech impairments. Speech deficiencies can be caused by a variety of factors, such as birth defects, injuries, or illnesses. A common speech deficiency is dysarthria, or interference with normal control of the speech mechanism. Diseases such as Parkinson's disease, multiple sclerosis, and bulbar palsy, as well as strokes and accidents, can cause dysarthria. In dysarthria, speech may be slurred or otherwise difficult to understand because of lack of ability to produce speech sounds correctly, maintain good breath control, or coordinate the movements of the lips, tongue, palate, and larynx. Many of these patients can be helped by certain medications or by therapy from a trained speech pathologist.

Another common speech problem results from the removal of the larynx secondary to throat cancer or other conditions. Such individuals can usually learn to speak again either by learning esophageal speech or by using an electronic device. However, you must be sensitive to these patients, since they sound "different." Many people realize that they sound different and may make other people feel uncomfortable. Thus, they may shy away from interacting with others.

To overcome speech barriers, many patients write notes to their pharmacist or use sign language as a means of communicating. Some pharmacists have responded to this need by providing writing pads for patients and even learning how to sign along with the patient.

APHASIA

A group of patients with related speech difficulties are those who suffer from aphasia after a stroke or another adverse event. Aphasia is a complex problem that may result, to varying degrees, in the reduced ability to understand what others are saying and to express oneself. Some patients may have no speech, whereas others may have only mild difficulties in recalling names or words. Others may have problems putting words in their proper order in a sentence. Speech may be limited to short phrases or single words, or smaller words are left out so that the sentence reads like a telegram. The ability to understand oral directions, to read, to write, and to deal with numbers may also be disturbed. Fortunately for some patients, their communication ability can be improved after extensive therapy. However, improvements are often seen in small increments.

Aphasic patients usually have normal hearing acuity; shouting at them will not help. Their problems are due to lack of comprehension; they are not hard of hearing, stubborn, or inattentive. Until you are aware of the extent of language impairment, avoid complex conversations. You need to be patient with these individuals when discussing their medications. Many times, they get frustrated with their situation because they know what they want to say but cannot say it. Also, it takes longer to communicate with them, since they may hear the word but may not immediately recall the meaning of it. Patience is also needed, since you may be tempted to fill in the word or phrase for aphasic patients. It is best to let them try to communicate. If they are unsuccessful after a few attempts, help them by supplying a few words in multiple-choice fashion and letting them select the word they desire. Aphasic patients often feel isolated and may withdraw from social interactions. Thus, they should be encouraged to interact with other people. Most appreciate being included in a conversation even if only to listen.

Some aphasic patients have difficulty reading. The difficulty is not one of visual acuity but rather of comprehending written language. Some have severe dyslexia and cannot read at all; others can read single words with comprehension but cannot read sentences. Patients with dyslexia may not be able to write notes to you. Dyslexia is not a physical disability but rather the inability to recall or form conventional written symbols.

Many aphasic patients retain certain automatic responses and may appear to be able to communicate very well. They may be able to count to 10 but not to count 4 items placed in front of them. They can name the days of the week, but cannot tell you that Tuesday comes before Thursday. They may be able to function effectively only in repetitive situations. Usually, their automatic speech skills are within socially acceptable limits, but sometimes patients utter profanities that may embarrass both listeners and patients themselves. Patients are not displaying anger or other displeasures when they curse, but rather are using automatic speech and are unable to inhibit these responses. You will probably be challenged when counseling aphasic patients and getting feedback may be difficult, but you should at least make an attempt, since they may benefit from the experience. Many times it is best to counsel other people who are caring for aphasic patients, but do not exclude patients from this experience.

Patients with Disabilities

One cannot anticipate all the various types of patients you will be interacting with during your career, but many will have disabilities that must be considered. In addition, there is a wide spectrum of how patients are able to cope with their disabilities. On one end of the spectrum, patients may be coping so well that their disability is hardly noticeable, while on the other end, their disability may severely affect their ability to access care and communicate with you. The key is to be sensitive to their unique needs. As many disabled individuals would say, "Don't treat me as a disability, treat me as an individual with a disability; in other words, treat me as an individual first." Using common sense and being sensitive to individual needs would be good practices to follow. Due to some disabilities, you may need to interact with the patient's caregiver rather than the patient. As discussed later in the chapter, this necessary approach presents a variety of communication issues.

WHEELCHAIR-BOUND PATIENTS

Access issues are paramount when caring for wheelchair-bound patients. The Americans with Disabilities Act (ADA) has specific guidelines regarding access to health care environments that would be applicable to pharmacies. Unfortunately, many pharmacy practice settings, including hospital, clinic, and community sites, are not readily accessible to these individuals. Entrances and aisles are often not wide enough, counters are too high, and pharmacists may not be visible to wheelchair-bound patients.

When talking with patients in wheelchairs, it is important to realize that you may be talking down to them. Although they may be used to having people hovering over them, it is best to talk on the same eye level, if it is not too awkward. Patients appreciate any efforts to minimize the distance between you and them without causing increased attention to the fact that they are in a wheelchair. You should watch patients' nonverbal messages to monitor whether they are comfortable during the communication process. You may need to adjust your location or approach if they appear to be straining to hear or do not seem satisfied with the communication environment.

LEARNING-DISABLED PATIENTS

Patients with learning disabilities are especially challenging since you do not want to treat them differently, but at the same time you want to make sure they can comprehend the critical information you provide, including how to take the medicine, proper storage requirements, or what side effects to monitor. You must develop tact in approaching these patient education situations. You may have to repeat key information or use a variety of analogies to make your point. In addition, you should not get frustrated if the patient does not seem to get the main points. Some pharmacists have developed effective written materials that are easy to understand and are targeted to an appropriate reading level. Unfortunately, most available literature is written on the 10th to 12th grade level, which is too complex for many learning-disabled patients. For many patients, you may also have to work with the patient's caregiver to make sure information is transmitted correctly and used appropriately. If the patient and caregiver are both present, make sure you speak to the patient, not just to the caregiver, to get them involved with the situation as much as possible.

HOMEBOUND PATIENTS

The key to communicating with homebound patients is to work with patients' caregivers when they visit the pharmacy to verify that information is transmitted correctly and used appropriately. Clear, concise written information is essential in these situations. It is critical to review this information with the caregiver to make sure key points are highlighted and are eventually discussed with the patient. Communication over the phone or Internet may also be possible (see Chapter 7 for advice on how to conduct an effective telephone interview). Many homebound patients can use the Internet and thus you may be able to communicate with them via e-mail.

The use of social networks has increased dramatically in recent years. In fact, the Pew Research Center (2010) reports that in 2010, 72% of all adults were texting messages using cell phones, making it a useful tool to "stay in touch" with homebound patients. You can also recommend links to appropriate Web sites for relevant information for the patient. It is very rare that pharmacists visit homebound patients, but patients and their caregivers certainly appreciate these visits. In addition, some health insurance companies will pay for pharmacy home visits, especially if they are linked to providing delivery and monitoring of special medication (e.g., home infusion).

Terminally Ill Patients

Most individuals, including pharmacists, find it somewhat difficult to interact with terminally ill patients. People typically feel uncomfortable discussing the topic of death and are uncertain about what to say; they do not want to say the "wrong" thing or upset patients. Yet most terminally ill patients need supportive relationships from family members, friends, and pharmacists.

Pharmacists are becoming increasingly important in the care of terminally ill patients owing to the complex nature of cancer therapy and pain management and to their increased involvement on oncology teams in hospitals and other institutions. By the same token, more community-based pharmacists and their staffs are getting involved because of the deinstitutionalization of cancer treatment and the evolution of home health care as a popular option for many patients. More importantly, pharmacists may be the only health professionals in their community who are readily accessible to patients and families. In addition, more patients are receiving palliative care at home. Palliative care seeks to comfort patients and to keep them pain-free, which helps address physical, as well as the psychological, emotional, and spiritual, needs of the patient. A key component of palliative care is effective communication between patients, pharmacists, and other health care providers. Managing these unique needs requires strong communication skills; thus, you should be ready, professionally and emotionally, to interact with these patients.

The key is to "meet the patients where they are" in their understanding of their condition and/or stage of adjustment. For example, one patient may be denying the existence of his illness while another might be angry or depressed about his situation. You would approach these two situations differently. The key is to ask open-ended questions, such as "How are you doing today?" or "How are things going?" to determine patient willingness to discuss the situation with you. You should not assume that patients do not want to talk about it. Even if patients do not respond initially, they at least realize that you are indicating you are willing to talk; thus, they may open up at a later time. In addition, you should not "push" patients who are in denial or angry to change their perceptions or feelings. Acceptance of whatever patients feel regardless of the coping strategies they use is an important aspect of caring.

Before interacting with terminally ill patients, be aware of your own feelings about death and interacting with terminally ill patients. Do you typically avoid conversations with these patients? Do they remind you of someone close to you who struggles with a terminal illness? Being aware of your feelings will help you assist these patients. You should realize that you can handle some situations yourself, whereas other cases should be referred to others for assistance. Many pharmacists have found that just being honest about their feelings improves their interaction with terminally ill patients. Just by saying "I don't know what to say right now. Tell me how I can help you?" or "I feel so helpless. Is there anything I can do for you?" seems to communicate concern for patients and gives them a chance to share their concerns as well. As in any type of patient interaction, the degree of involvement depends on your relationship with the patient. You will be more open with some patients than with others. It is also important to implicitly or explicitly set limits on what you can do for the patient. You must communicate your concern without raising the patient's expectations that you can assist in all areas of the patient's life, such as providing financial advice or preparing a will. Many terminally ill patients realize they make other people feel uncomfortable. Thus, they tend to avoid certain interactions. However, if you can express your uneasiness or your frustration about not knowing how to help them at the same time that you express concern for them, patients will typically feel more at ease and more willing to express their own feelings.

You may also come in contact with family members who will probably have special needs themselves. Research has shown that family members go through the same types of stages (denial, bargaining, anger, depression, and acceptance) that dying patients go through; they also need support and, at times, drug therapy (Kübler-Ross, 2005). Thus, you should be prepared to deal with the various emotions associated with each stage. In addition, Kübler-Ross and others have found that many individuals do not enter all stages and often move back and forth between various levels of denial and acceptance. Therefore, you need to listen closely to family members to determine their specific needs.

In summary, communicating with terminally ill patients and their families is extremely important. You should not avoid talking with them unless you sense they do not want to talk about their illness. Not interacting with them only contributes further to their social isolation and may reaffirm the idea that talking about death with others should be avoided.

Patients with Sexually Communicated Infections

As a pharmacist, you will probably be working with patients who have a variety of sensitive health issues related to sexually communicated infections such as HIV or gonorrhea. Not only are these patients dealing with serious diseases, they are also dealing with the social stigmas that often accompany their condition. Typically, they do have a unique set of needs that should be recognized and addressed. Therefore, you may have to adjust their thinking about these diseases. In any case, you should use some of the strategies outlined in the previous text, such as using open-ended questions to determine patient receptivity to interaction. It also may be important to determine if patients have adequate support systems, since relationships with family and friends may be strained because of the social stigma. It is important to reflect on what your role should be in assisting patients. You may be called on to refer the patient to an appropriate source of social assistance and support. You may also need to supply additional triage or problem-solving support when others are not providing it. The key is to identify what the patient's needs are and what services you can provide or referrals you can make to best meet these needs.

In regard to patients with HIV, many have trouble dealing with their own identity as the disease progresses. In many cases, dealing with HIV or AIDS has physical components (i.e., weight loss, lack of energy), but also psychological and sociological aspects (i.e., becoming more dependent on others, fear of dying, dealing with a chronic disease). Some patients may be wrestling with a lot of issues and may need assistance sorting things out. Patients must also deal with misinformation and inaccurate perceptions about HIV and AIDS. People around them may not understand various aspects of the disease or its treatment. It is hoped that you are not included in this misinformed group. You must keep up with the latest literature, since many patients monitor what is being researched and publicized.

Patients with Mental Health Problems

Many pharmacists admit they have difficulty in communicating with patients with mental health disorders. Some pharmacists feel they do not know what to say to mental health patients. They are afraid to say the wrong thing or something that might cause an emotional outburst by the patient in the pharmacy. Unfortunately, certain stereotypes about mental illness and patients with these disorders tend to inhibit communication. People in general, as well as many pharmacists, have certain misconceptions about mental illness. We tend to categorize people based on images from the media or beliefs we have formed about how "crazy" people act. Our reluctance is also reinforced by the fact that some patients indeed act "different." They may have awkward body and facial movements (possibly due to their medications). Some are chronic cigarette smokers and have poor hygienic habits. They may make what we consider to be bizarre statements. They may not establish good eye contact, which may make us even more uncomfortable. By the same token, many mental health patients may be reluctant to interact with other individuals for a variety of reasons. First, they may have a poor self-concept and may be insecure about interacting with others. They may also realize they have a condition that makes other people uncomfortable. This societal stigma about mental illness may make them avoid social interactions. In some cases, patients may be paranoid about dealing with other people, especially health care professionals. Thus, your attempts to communicate may find initial patient resistance.

Some pharmacists are also unsure of how much information to provide to such patients about their condition and treatment. Many times it is unclear what patients understand about their condition and what their physicians have told them. Once again, open-ended questions are good tools to determine the level of patient understanding before you counsel them about their medications. Examples include "What has the doctor told you about this medication?" or "This drug can be used for different things. What has your physician said?" Asking open-ended questions also helps you determine patient cognitive functioning. That is, are they able to comprehend what you are saying, and can they articulate their concerns to you? If not, you may have to communicate through a caregiver.

Some pharmacists may be reluctant to distribute written information to patients receiving psychotropic medications for fear that patients may misinterpret the information. A related concern is that many psychotropic medications are used for nonmental health disorders, such as imipramine for bed-wetting or diazepam for muscle spasms. Thus, the written material may not be relevant to the patient's condition and may only cause alarm. It is important that you carefully screen all materials for their relevance to the individual patient before distribution and that you attempt to verbally reinforce the information to ensure a better understanding by the patient.

Pharmacists interacting with patients with mental disorders must address a more fundamental ethical issue: Should patients with mental disorders be allowed the same level of information regarding their drug treatment and the same type of informed consent as patients with nonpsychiatric disorders? Does the uniqueness of having a mental illness versus a physical illness preclude these patients from knowing more about the effects (both positive and negative) of their drugs? Do we withhold certain information that would be given to a nonpsychiatric patient? Obviously, each situation must be evaluated individually, and many times in consultation with the patient's physician and caregiver. However, the issue is raised here because the way you deal with these questions affects how you communicate with mental health patients. In many situations, trusting relationships develop among patients, mental health practitioners, and pharmacists. In these cases, pharmacists can be key members of the patient's care management team. Regardless, you should be aware of the ethical responsibility to provide patients with accurate information in a way that meets their need to understand their treatments. Only with compelling reasons can health professionals ignore the principle that patients have the right to information about their treatment.

Patients with mental illness typically need multiple contacts to establish trusting relationships. However, you should realize this may never happen and your interactions may always be "different" compared with your relationships with other patients. These differences should be handled the same way that you deal with other unique individuals discussed in previous sections. Differences should not stop you from trying to interact with these patients. However, the potential communication problems may require you to be innovative in developing strategies to overcome them.

Suicidal Patients

A patient who has been taking hydrocodone for the past 9 months due to severe chronic back pain approaches you in your ambulatory care pharmacy and says, "Boy, dealing with this chronic pain is no picnic. How much of this stuff would it take to kill someone?" What would go through your mind? What would you say? You might consider the possibility that this patient is suicidal. However, you might not be sure. How can you tell whether the patient's question represents a cry for help or just talk? If you indeed perceive this patient to be suicidal, how confident would you be that you could communicate effectively with him? How would you approach this situation?

Before discussing how you may respond, it might be helpful to first identify some of the myths surrounding suicide that may prevent you from offering help to this potentially suicidal person.

Myth 1. "People who talk about committing suicide just want attention and do not actually kill themselves." In fact, the majority of individuals who commit suicide have given warnings about their intent. Their clear statements or more subtle hints about wanting to end it all or feelings that others would be better off if they disappeared should be seen as a "cry for help." They want someone to recognize their need and respond.

Myth 2. "People who have seriously attempted or actually committed suicide wanted to die." Evidence is that individuals in a suicidal crisis are motivated by a desire to escape extreme psychological pain and feelings of despair. Their thinking has become so distorted that they believe the only way to escape the pain is to die. The cognitive constriction also leads them to lose hope that relief from their suffering is possible or effective treatment is possible.

Myth 3. "Suicidal risk is greatest when individuals are in the depths of a major depressive episode." Surprisingly, suicides often follow a period when people seem to be coming out of their depressed states. Family and friends are thus shocked because they thought the worst was over.

Myth 4. "Asking depressed individuals whether they are suicidal is dangerous because it may get them to consider suicide when they hadn't been thinking of it before." The fact is that you will not put suicidal thoughts into people's minds who have not been considering suicide. Asking about suicide will likely provide a sense that you care about them. If the patient who asks about the lethal dose of hydrocodone is not suicidal, he will clarify the reason for his question. If he is depressed or in despair (which often accompanies chronic, severe pain), your question may provide an opening for him to tell you what he is feeling. You can then provide the empathy, support, and information on sources of help that he needs.

Myth 5. "Once a person decides to commit suicide, there is nothing anyone can do to stop him." The reality is that the acute crisis is short-lived. However, effective treatment of the underlying depression is necessary to prevent future crises. Further information on the myths surrounding suicide is available from the organizations listed in Box 10.1.

When faced with someone you think may be suicidal, you must have the courage to talk about your concerns. Say to the patient who asks about the lethal dose of hydrocodone, "I'm concerned about the reason behind the question. Are you thinking about killing yourself?" If the question is a cry for help, you have provided the opening for the patient to admit to needing help. Stay calm. Listen with empathy. Express your caring for the patient and your desire to help. Avoid arguing with him or trying to get him to justify why he feels the despair he obviously feels. Don't discuss your own values or moral objections to suicide. Have someone stay with the individual until he is under professional care. Be familiar with sources of help in your community.

Make a note in the patient's profile about their statements and your conversations with the patient in case another colleague deals with the patient during the next encounter. This is especially important when patients are taking medications that exacerbate depression. You and your colleagues need to monitor these situations and respond appropriately. If you are not sure what help is available, call the crisis intervention or suicide prevention help lines that are prominently listed in the front of most telephone books. Help and advice are also available through the National Suicide Prevention Lifeline at 1-800-273-8255. Various Web sites provide information on recognizing suicidal intent and advice on responding to someone in crisis (see Box 10.1).

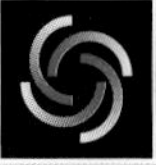

Box 10.1 Helpful Web Sites for Suicide Prevention

- The National Center for Injury Prevention and Control at the Centers for Disease Control and Prevention: www.cdc.gov/injury/index.html
- The American Association of Suicidology: www.suicidology.org
- The American Foundation for Suicide Prevention: www.afsp.org
- The Suicide Prevention Resource Center: www.sprc.org

Patients with Low Health Literacy

Low health literacy is a pervasive problem that impedes the ability of many patients to understand information you provide about their medications. Health literacy is the ability to "read, understand and act on healthcare information" (AMA Ad Hoc Committee on Health Literacy, 1999). Studies have found that 90 million Americans have limited health literacy (Nielsen-Bohlman et al., 2004). About 34% of English-speaking and 54% of Spanish-speaking American adults have marginal literacy. The average reading level in these populations is eighth grade, while most health information is written at the 12th grade level. About 15% of patients with literacy problems are foreign-born and 5% are learning disabled, which means that 80% of the population with literacy issues were born in this country and do not have a documented learning disability.

To illustrate the extent of the problem, one study found that 42% of patients could not read and comprehend directions for administering a medication on an empty stomach (Williams et al., 1995). At the same time, health care professionals are largely unaware of the extent of the problem in society and in their own population of patients. Persons with limited ability to read and comprehend information are frequently embarrassed and fail to disclose this fact to health care providers. Due to the strong stigma associated with reading problems, many patients will make excuses or try to conceal the fact that they have trouble reading. Many patients with literacy issues have average IQs and function well in daily life, so detection is difficult. Unfortunately, health care providers typically fail to assess patients' understanding of written information provided to them (see Chapter 8 for additional information regarding reading level assessment of written materials you provide to patients).

The key to this dilemma is that poor health literacy is directly linked to patient safety. If patients cannot understand the material, they are in danger of therapeutic misadventures and medication errors. The issue is so important that the U.S. Congress has proclaimed October as Health Literacy Month (see *A Quick Guide to Health Literacy* available at: www.health.gov/communication/literacy/quickguide/).

As far as strategies to deal with this issue, some research has found that providing pictures along with simple written instructions can improve comprehension of key medication instructions (Morrow et al., 1998). The United States Pharmacopeia (USP) has developed 81 pictograms that illustrate common medication instructions and precautions. These graphic images can be downloaded from the USP Web site (www.usp.org) and used by health care professionals to supplement written instructions for low-literate or non-English-speaking patients. In addition, the American Medical Association Foundation has produced a Health Literacy Introductory Kit for health care providers describing the scope of the health literacy problem and suggesting ways to overcome barriers to communication (www.ama-assn.org). Hardin (2005) suggests that, among other things, pharmacists should have their patients summarize instructions to ensure accurate transmission of information. See Box 10.2.

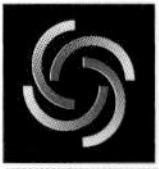

Box 10.2 Relevant Health Literacy Web Sites

1. National Library of Medicines current bibliographies on health literacy: www.nlm.nih.gov/archive//20061214/pubs/cbm/hliteracy.html. Retrieved September 2010.
2. National Institute for Literacy: lincs.ed.gov/
   The National Institute for Literacy provides national leadership regarding literacy, coordinates literacy services and policy, and serves as a national resource for adult education and literacy programs. It also disseminates information on scientifically based reading research pertaining to children, youth, and adults as well as information about development and implementation of classroom reading programs based on the research. Retrieved September 2010.
3. National Center for Cultural Competence (NCCC): nccc.georgetown.edu/
   The National Center for Cultural Competence's mission is to increase the capacity of health and mental health programs to design, implement, and evaluate culturally and linguistically competent service delivery systems. Retrieved September 2010.
4. Literacy on Line: www.literacyonline.org/
   A non-profit organization interested in improving health literacy. Retrieved September 2010.

Cultural Competence

As mentioned earlier, you may be working with patients who are different than yourself. Some of these differences relate to culture and ethnic background. Thus, you must have sensitivity to the cultural differences in your diverse patient environment. This will become even more critical in the future since, according to the projected demographic changes in the United States, our country will become even more diverse. It is beyond the scope of this chapter to describe all the various cultures within the United States and their related beliefs about health care and medication therapy, but a few general guidelines are offered to assist you in developing your cultural competence and enhancing your ability to work with patients from diverse backgrounds (see Box 10.3). First, you may want to examine the cultural makeup of your practice catchment area. What are the predominant ethnic groups in the neighborhoods surrounding your practice site? What are their overall feelings about the accessibility and quality of health care? What is their trust level regarding health care in general and medication management specifically? You may want to speak with community leaders to assess general community beliefs. Together you may be able to develop strategies for interacting with various groups. Learning more about these cultures is a challenging but necessary task.

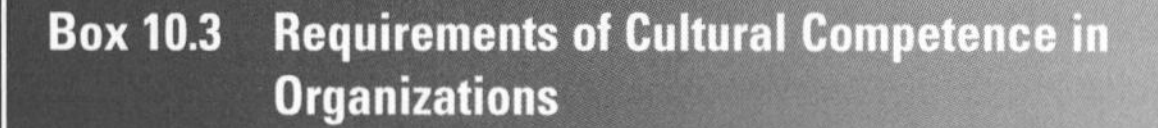

Box 10.3 Requirements of Cultural Competence in Organizations

- Have a defined set of values and principles, and demonstrate behaviors, attitudes, policies, and structures that enable members at the organization to work effectively cross-culturally.
- Have the capacity to (1) value diversity, (2) conduct self-assessment, (3) manage the dynamics of difference, (4) acquire and institutionalize cultural knowledge, and (5) adapt to diversity and the cultural contexts of the communities the organization serves.
- Incorporate the above in all aspects of policy making, administration, practice, and service delivery and systematically involve consumers, key stakeholders, and communities.
- Develop programs to identify and understand the needs and help-seeking behaviors of individuals and families served by the organization.

Source: National Center for Cultural Competence, 2004. Retrieved September 2010 from nccc.georgetown.edu.

Since various cultures speak a variety of languages, one issue that may arise is your ability to communicate with patients who do not speak English or have marginal English skills. As described in the interviewing chapter (Chapter 7), it is important to assess your patient's ability to comprehend or speak the language you are using. If language appears to be a significant barrier to communication, you must use one of the strategies discussed earlier, such as using a staff member who speaks the patient's primary language or using written material they can understand.

In looking at broader public health issues, a better understanding of culture may lead to resolving some of the many documented health disparity issues. Research has found that many minority populations do not receive the same level of care as other groups within the United States (Sicat and Hill, 2005). Thus, they are at a disadvantage and often do not receive appropriate care. These disparities tend to lead to a variety of chronic health problems. A better understanding of the barriers to care could lead to strategies for improving access to health care. You should be aware that several governmental and private foundation programs have been established to assist health care providers in improving health disparity issues. Some of these programs' Web sites are listed on page 175. Fortunately, funds may be available to assist you in caring for certain groups of patients.

In summary, cultural competence is a developmental process that evolves over an extended period. Individuals and organizations are currently at various levels of awareness, knowledge, and skills along the cultural competence continuum. The key is to be sensitive to the differences in beliefs and behaviors and the disparities related to access to care within your diverse patient populations. At the same time, you should not stereotype individuals based on their ethnic background, as discussed earlier. The best strategy is to ask open-ended questions to determine what exactly patients feel about certain elements within their health care.

Caregivers

Several special communication problems arise when you and your staff must interact with patient caregivers rather than with patients themselves. Caregivers can be people who take care of older adults with chronic conditions, parents who take care of children during acute or chronic illnesses, family members, friends, or hired assistants. In general, the number of these caregivers will probably increase in the future, since there has been an increased effort to shift patient care from hospitals to home care. Dealing with caregivers requires specific strategies, since you cannot communicate directly with patients and thus cannot determine whether they received your intended message. It is also difficult to assess patient adherence with medication regimens and to offer support and encouragement to patients regarding their medication treatment.

When dealing with caregivers, certain areas should be addressed. First, caregivers need to understand the patient's condition and treatment and how to communicate specific instructions to the patient. Caregivers must also understand how to monitor patient therapeutic response to a specific medication, how to monitor for adverse drug events, and how to report any suspicious events. They should be instructed about the importance of good nutrition and fluid intake for certain types of patients. They must be reminded about the refill status of medications and when their physicians need to be contacted. Caregivers should be encouraged to contact you if they have questions or the patient has questions.

Written information about the medication is essential, since the message should be delivered to patients. A follow-up phone call to patients may also be necessary to make sure messages were received and to reinforce key points regarding drug therapy. Many pharmacists use medication reminder systems (i.e., drug calendars, weekly medication containers) to help caregivers keep track of medications.

In addition, you should develop a special sensitivity to caregivers and should not merely view them as someone picking up the medication. Many times, caregivers have special needs themselves. They may be under a lot of stress trying to care for the patient at home. They may have careers and other activities outside the home and may be financially strained as well. Serious depression has been found in almost one-fourth of the individuals caring for the homebound elderly. In some situations, the caregivers may be patients themselves with their own medical problems. One of the fastest-growing segments of our population is the group of people over 65 with parents in their 80s and 90s. Thus, two generations of patients with health problems may be living in the same home.

You should respond empathetically to caregivers and try to understand some of their personal problems. As mentioned earlier, pharmacists are often the most accessible health care professionals in the community and may be the only consistent contact caregivers have with the health care network. You should be aware of the caregiver's nonverbal messages and must not be afraid to ask, "What is on your mind?" You should also be aware of support groups in the community that could assist caregivers, such as local hospice organizations for terminally ill patients at home or respite care services to ease caregiver burdens. You should realize that dealing with a terminal illness or other devastating disease may reduce family members' ability to communicate with each other and health care providers. Caregivers have so much stress in their daily lives that it is often difficult for them to express needs related to their own well-being.

Summary

You will always be challenged by situations needing special attention within pharmacy practice. Although the groups discussed in this chapter do not represent the entire universe of patients with special communication needs, they do reflect groups that deserve special consideration. The following chapter addresses another special group of patients—children who are dealing with health issues. With all patients, you need to first recognize patients with special communication needs and then develop effective strategies to overcome specific barriers to the communication process.

REVIEW QUESTIONS

1. **What impact does aging have on learning, memory, and recall?**
2. **Is there such a thing as a generation gap when counseling patients? If so, explain.**
3. **What is aphasia, and how can you communicate with a patient who has it?**
4. **Describe your feelings about the terminally ill and how you could best communicate with them.**
5. **What are some of the special communication problems that arise from interactions with caregivers?**

REVIEW CASES

REVIEW CASE STUDY 10.1

Nellie Curtis, age 83, has been a member of a large managed-care plan since its inception in 1985. She became a member as part of her husband's employee benefits package when his employer converted shortly after his retirement. She has always had her prescriptions filled at the clinic pharmacy run by her plan. On this occasion, she enters the pharmacy to pick up refills for two of her medications, a diuretic and a digitalis glycoside. Marcus, the pharmacist, greets Nellie:

Marcus: Hello, Nellie! I bet you are having a good day today.

Nellie: Not really, but why are you so sure?

Marcus: Because with all this rain we've been having it's gotta be good for the crops and making the grass green.

Nellie: Well, I guess so.

Marcus: Here are your medicines. Let's see, you take one of each once a day, except the little white one is every other day. Right?

Nellie: Yup, I think you've got it.

Marcus: You have been on this stuff a long time, haven't you?

Nellie: Yup, 'bout a decade.

Marcus: You're not having any problems with them, are you?

Nellie: Well, I mustn't be, I'm still around, aren't I? Say, why all the questions?

Marcus: It's our new policy to talk to people. There is a law that says we need to talk more to customers.

Nellie: It's about time!

Marcus: Well, Nellie, y'all have a good one.

1. How could Marcus have better prepared this elderly patient for a counseling encounter?
2. How should he have established a more respectful relationship?
3. How could Marcus have assessed and responded to any of Mrs. Curtis' needs related to sight, hearing, or memory loss?
4. What simple sentences could Marcus have used to ensure Mrs. Curtis' understanding of how and why she takes her medicines?
5. Some of Marcus' comments appeared to be leading, restrictive, and judgmental in nature. Rewrite Marcus' dialogue to let Mrs. Curtis respond with items that are important to her.

REVIEW CASE STUDY 10.2

A patient who looks somewhat depressed approaches the prescription counter and says, "Boy, I can't believe what is happening to me. I went to the doctor because I was feeling kind of low. She gave me a prescription for Ambien (zolpidem). It certainly helps me sleep, but I still feel depressed. Did you ever wonder if life was worth the hassle?"

1. How would you respond to this person?
2. What special needs does this patient seem to have?
3. What is your role in this situation?

REFERENCES

AMA Ad Hoc Committee on Health Literacy. Health Literacy: Report of the Council on Scientific Affairs. *Journal of the American Medical Association* 281:552–557, 1999.

Hardin, LR. Counseling patients with low health literacy. *American Journal of Hospital Pharmacy* 62:364–365, 2005.

Kübler-Ross, E. *On Grief and Grieving: Finding the Meaning of Grief through the Five Stages of Loss*. New York, NY: Simon & Schuster, 2005.

Morrow DG, Hier CM, Menard WE, Leirer VO. Icons improve older and younger adults' comprehension of medication information. *Journal of Gerontology* 53:P240–P254, 1998.

Nielsen-Bohlman L, Panzer AM, Kindig DA (eds.). *Health Literacy: A Prescription to End Confusion*. Washington, DC: National Academy Press, 2004.

Pew Research Center, Internet and American Life Project, May 2010. Available at http://pewinternet.org/Reports/2010/Cell-Phones-and-American-Adults.aspx. Accessed September, 2010.

Sicat BL, Hill LH. Enhancing student knowledge about the prevalence and consequences of low health literacy. *American Journal of Pharmaceutical Education* 69: article 62, 2005.

Williams MU, Parker RM, Baker DW, et al. Inadequate functional health literacy among patients at two public hospitals. *Journal of the American Medical Association* 274:1677–1682, 1995.

RECOMMENDED READINGS

American Medical Association. Good care of the dying patient. *Journal of the American Medical Association* 275:474–478, 1994.

American Psychological Association. *Guidelines for Psychological Practice with Older Adults*. Available at http://www.apa.org/practice/guidelines/older-adults.pdf. Accessed September 30, 2010.

Brookshire RH. *An Introduction to Neurogenic Communication Disorders*. St. Louis, MO: Mosby-Year Book, 1992.

Damasio AR. Aphasia. *New England Journal of Medicine* 326:531–539, 1992.

Osborne, H. *Health Literacy from A to Z: Practical Ways to Communicate Your Health Message*. Sudbury, MA: Jones and Bartlett Publishers, 2005.

Osborn H. In Other Words, Using Text Messages to Improve Medication Adherence. *On Call Magazine* September 18, 2008.

Shah MB, King S, Patel AS. Intercultural disposition and communication competence of future pharmacists. *American Journal of Pharmaceutical Education* 68: article 111, 2004.

Youmans SL, Schillinger D. Functional health literacy and medication use: The pharmacist's role. *Annals of Pharmacotherapy* 37:1726–1729, 2003.

CHAPTER

11

Communicating with Children about Medicines

BETSY L. SLEATH AND PATRICIA J. BUSH

Overview

Children are important consumers of medicines. Communicating with children is different from communicating with adults in two distinct ways. First, communication with children about medicines typically involves three people: a health care provider, a child, and the child's parent. Second, children being educated about medicines need to be educated at a level that is appropriate for their cognitive developmental levels. This chapter discusses the following: (a) the need for educating children and their parents about medicines, (b) the importance of using a patient-centered style with children and parents, (c) how to understand the cognitive developmental level of a child, (d) strategies for communicating with and empowering children at different ages about their medicines, (e) what children want to know about medicines at different ages, and (f) assessing family barriers to medicine adherence.

Need for Educating Children and Their Parents about Medicines

If you refer to the interpersonal communication model in Chapter 2, you will see that when you communicate about children's medicines, you are potentially sending messages to two receivers—a child and a parent. Ranelli et al. (2000) found in a study of Wyoming pharmacists that pharmacists reported considerable contact with children and their families and that most pharmacists (87%) reported filling prescriptions for children daily. However, when the pharmacists were asked whether they communicated directly with children, 33% claimed they did so most of the time, 32% reported doing so some of the time, and 35% reported that they rarely communicated with children. However, most pharmacists reported they thought children should become more active participants in their medicine use.

When parents come into the pharmacy to purchase prescription or over-the-counter (OTC) medicines for their child, it is important to educate the child as well as the parent about the medicine. In addition to educating the child, an advantage to communicating directly with the child is that you are more likely to speak at a level the parent will understand.

There is evidence that children do not receive much education about medicines from physicians or pharmacists. Ranelli et al. found that 83% of pharmacists reported that physicians give little information about medicines to children despite their need. Sleath et al. (2010) found that 87% of 320 children reported a problem or concern in using their asthma medicines. Approximately 40% of children reported side effects and a similar percentage stated it was hard to understand the directions on their medicines; 60% reported that it was hard to remember when to take their medicines. Menacker et al. (1999) interviewed 85 healthy public school children from grades kindergarten through eighth grade in focus groups and found that most of the children reported learning about medicines from their mothers. The children reported that physicians and pharmacists played a limited role in educating them about medicines. Hämeen-Anttila et al. (2005) found that fourth-graders were most interested in learning about how medicines work, how to avoid adverse reactions, and abuse of medicines. Most of these fourth-graders reported that they would like to ask the doctor or pharmacist a question about medicine, but they reported never doing so. These results suggest that pharmacists need to encourage children to ask questions about their medicines. The easiest way to do this is to say to a child: “Nearly everyone who gets a medicine has questions about it, including grownups. I bet you have questions, too. Can you tell me a question you have about your medicines?”

There is also evidence that pharmacists need to educate children about OTC medicines. One study found that 36% of 10- to 14-year-old children had self-medicated the last time they had taken a medicine (Sloand and Vesey, 2001). Bush and Davidson (1982) examined the amount of autonomy that 64 urban children in kindergarten through sixth grades exhibited when it came to medicine taking. They found that nearly 20% of the children, more often older children and those in less economically advantaged neighborhoods, reported purchasing OTC medicines by themselves. The researchers also found that, of the children who reported taking a medicine “yesterday or today,” 75% said they took the medicine by themselves, and 40% said they got the medicine by themselves from somewhere in the house. In a follow-up study of 300 urban schoolchildren in grades three through seven, 25% of the children reported purchasing an OTC

CASE STUDY 11.1

A father picked up an oral antibiotic suspension prescription for his son who had a severe infection. Due to the relatively high dose of the antibiotic and the need for a longer period of treatment, the father was given two bottles of antibiotic and was told to give one teaspoonful twice a day. When he reached home, he gave his son one teaspoonful from *both* bottles. Fortunately, the mother questioned this approach once she realized what was going on, called the pharmacy for clarification, and continued therapy at the appropriate level.

medicine independently and 37% reported picking up a prescription independently (Iannotti and Bush, 1992). Follow-up visits to pharmacies and places selling medicines confirmed that school-age children purchase OTC medicines and pick up prescriptions.

Pharmacists need to better educate parents about their children's medicines. Ranelli et al. (2000) found that 42% of pharmacists reported that physicians give parents little information about medicines. As a pharmacist, you need to make sure parents are informed about their children's medicines to prevent errors. If you think about the various strengths of infant and children's acetaminophen and ibuprofen that are available in pharmacies and the many different types of pediatric cough and cold products that are for sale, you can understand how parents can become confused. Case Study 11.1 describes an actual situation involving communication issues with parents.

Pharmacists need to assess what children know about their prescription and OTC medicines by using open-ended questions and then filling in the gaps with education for both parent and child. You may apply the principles you learned in Chapter 8 about building better patient understanding when interacting with parents and their children.

Importance of Using a Patient-Centered Interaction Style

It is important to use a patient-centered interaction style when communicating with parents and children about medicines. Unfortunately, the amount of research on pharmacist–parent–child communication has not been extensive (Ranelli et al., 2000). Therefore, to further understand why it is important to educate both parents and children, we need to examine some of the previous work on pediatrician–child–parent communication. A review of the literature by Tates and Meeuwesen (2001) concluded that children are not included as active participants in discussions concerning their health during visits with physicians. Wissow et al. (1998) examined physician–parent–child communication about asthma during emergency room visits and found that children took little part in discussions. However, the researchers did find that if physicians used a patient-centered style with children, this was associated with five times more talk with

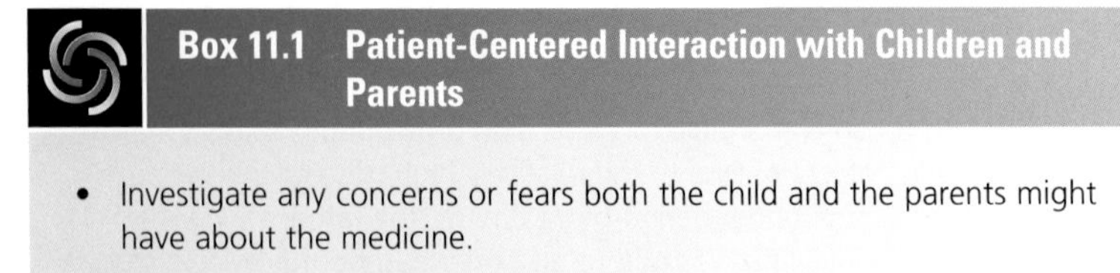

Box 11.1 Patient-Centered Interaction with Children and Parents

- Investigate any concerns or fears both the child and the parents might have about the medicine.
- Ask both the child and the parents about priorities for improved quality of life.
- If the child is on continued therapy, assess how well the child and the parents perceive the medicine is working.
- Offer to call the pediatrician to suggest possible changes in therapy if needed based on what you learn from the child and the parents.
- Ask both the child and the parents what questions they have about the medicine.
- Educate both the child and the parents about the medicine by communicating directly with the child when possible.

children and higher parent ratings of good care. A patient-centered style is one in which the health care provider seeks the child's opinions about treatment and empowers the child to seek information. The process of empowerment can be seen as building up knowledge, skills, and competencies, with participation a crucial element of this process (Kieffer, 1984; Rodwell, 1996).

Previous work in both adults and children has shown that patients are more adherent to medicine regimens and have better outcomes if they are taught about their disease and included in treatment decisions (Kelly and Scott, 1990; Street et al., 1993; Stewart, 1995; Stewart et al., 2000; Adams et al., 2001). See Box 11.1 for ways to use a patient-centered interaction style.

Understanding the Cognitive Developmental Level of a Child

A discussion of the developmental level of children will help you understand how to educate children at different ages and developmental levels about their medicines. Children progress through four stages as they develop cognitive skills. The classification of the four stages is based on the work of Piaget (1932), who examined the development of thinking skills in children. The four stages of cognitive development are (a) the sensory motor stage, (b) the preoperational stage, (c) the concrete operational stage, and (d) the formal operational stage. It is very important to remember that not all children pass through the stages at the same rate.

The *sensory motor* stage lasts from birth to roughly 2 years of age. During this stage, all learning is centered around the child, and there is little connection to objects outside the self. Learning about medicines is not really possible in this stage. Learning about medicines does become possible in the later stages.

The *preoperational* stage lasts from about age 2 through 6 years. During this stage, children tend to consider only a single aspect of a situation and often engage in "magical" thinking. Their reasoning is connected to the concrete reality of the here and now. Cause-and-effect relationships are difficult for preoperational children to understand, so children at this stage will see no connection between their own health and health-related behaviors (e.g., taking a prescribed medicine) (Lau and Klepper, 1988).

The *concrete operational* stage lasts from about age 7 through 12 years. During this stage, children begin to distinguish between the internal and external world. They can use symbols to represent concrete objects and perform mental operations. They can focus on multiple aspects of a situation at one time, and they become problem solvers. However, situations are best presented to them in a concrete or observable manner (O'Brien and Bush, 1993). During this stage, children begin to understand that disease is preventable, and their understanding of health and illness incorporates internal physiological characteristics.

The *formal operational* stage typically is from age 13 through adulthood. As children move into adolescence, they become capable of hypothetical and abstract thought. They can reason logically, and their understanding of how one gets sick becomes more realistic. Adolescents begin to develop increased awareness of degrees of illness as well as personal control of their health.

These stages can vary with the individual. However, it is generally accepted that, whereas individuals rarely think at a higher level than their age indicates, they often think at a lower level, and the level may be situation-dependent. Thus, for example, an adult may think "magically" about a health issue, "I caught a cold because I went out in the rain," but never about an issue related to his or employment.

You need to ask children open-ended questions when they come into the pharmacy. Closed-ended questions provide little information because a child will just answer yes or no. A child's answer to a pharmacist's open-ended questions should help reveal his or her cognitive level (O'Brien and Bush, 1993). After you determine a child's cognitive level, you can adapt how you communicate with him or her (see Box 11.2 for suggestions).

General Principles for Communicating with and Empowering Children

Some children as young as 3 or 4 years and most children by age 7 or 8 can actively participate in and contribute during visits with health care providers (Behrman and Vaughan, 1983; O'Brien and Bush, 1993). The following general strategies for communicating with children about medicines are adapted from Bush and Hämeen-Anttila (2009):

1. Attempt to communicate at the child's developmental level.
2. Tell the parent that you are going to talk with the child.
3. Start with some general questions about other things to get an idea of the child's developmental level.
4. Ask open-ended questions rather than questions requiring only a "yes" or "no" response so you can assess what the child understands.

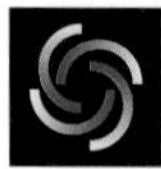

Box 11.2 Communication Strategies for Different Stages of Cognitive Development

PRE-OPERATIONAL STAGE (AGE 2 TO 7 YEARS)

Sample educational message: The medicine you'll get will go into your body and make your throat feel better. It will work only if you take it three times every day. Your mom will help you know when to take the medicine and when to stop taking the medicine. Be sure to use all the medicine, even if you think you're feeling better.

CONCRETE OPERATIONAL STAGE (AGE 7 TO 13 YEARS)

Sample educational message: This medicine will go into your body to help fight off the germs that are causing the infection in your throat. The medicine will work only if you take it three times a day until (date treatment should end). If you don't take it this way, the infection might come back. So keep taking the medicine, even if you think you're feeling better. Work with your mom or dad, so you both know you have taken the medicine at the right times.

FORMAL OPERATIONS STAGE (AGE 13 YEARS TO ADULTHOOD)

Sample educational message: The medicine you're getting will go into your system to help your immune system fight off bacteria that are causing your infection. You have strep throat, which is when a particular form of bacteria causes an irritation in your throat. The medicine used to treat these bacteria is an antibiotic. You have to take it every 8 hours—that is, three times a day—for the next 10 days. If you don't do this, there is a chance you will be reinfected. Keep taking your medicine until it is gone, even if you think your throat is better.

Source: O'Brien R, Bush P. Helping children learn how to use medicines. *Office Nurse* 6:14–19, 1993.

5. Use simple declarative sentences for all children.
6. If the child uses a medicine device, such as a metered dose inhaler, ask the child to demonstrate how they use it and then demonstrate how to use it correctly if needed.
7. Ask the child whether he or she has questions for you. (Note: You can lead into this by telling the child a simple question that another child asked you.)
8. Ask the child to repeat what you say.
9. Augment verbal communication with written communication.
10. Don't give up. If you fail the first time, try again the next time.
11. Pay attention to nonverbal communication.

Nonverbal communication is very important to children. Children attend to and interpret nonverbal communication before they understand the meanings of words (Behrman and Vaughan, 1983). If you think about it, much of the communication between children and parents is nonverbal (e.g., hugs, sounds, gestures). Therefore, when you interact with children, you need to be aware of your facial expressions, tone of voice, and gestures (Behrman and Vaughan, 1983). Also, try to get down to their level so you will not be "talking down" to them.

Next, we are going to discuss specific communication strategies to use with children of different ages. We will assume that interactions with children typically begin once a child is about 2 years of age and has moved into the preoperational (sometimes called "magical thinking") stage of development. Accompanying Box 11.3 outlines what children of different ages have said they want to know about medicines (Bush, 1999).

Toddlers and Preschool Children

Although toddlers and preschool children may not be as actively involved in learning about medicines as older children, it is important to include them in discussions about their medicines. A good way to begin an encounter with toddlers and preschool children is to start with a simple friendly greeting and then do an enthusiastic but brief examination of one of the child's toys (Coulehan and Block, 1992). In Ranelli's study (2000), a pharmacist reported special tactics for dealing with children. "It's good to have an icebreaker for kids. I always have a stash of bouncy balls and do a 'magic trick.' Once one has gained their attention and confidence, giving instructions becomes much easier." At this age, it is important to begin educating children in simple terms as to what the medicine is for and why it is important to take it.

Another pharmacist in Ranelli's study commented on his son's diagnosis with asthma at age 3, "Even then he understood why the medicine was important and when he needed a puff. He was in charge of his inhalers from second grade on because he was too shy to go to the school nurse." At this age, you want the child to feel that taking medicines is important. However, you also want to emphasize that the child should not take medicines without permission from mom or dad. You could do something as simple as letting the child put a label on the prescription. This way the child will know it is his or her own medicine and will also relieve the anxiety that young children have about mistakenly taking an adult's medicine (see Box 11.3). Educating children as young as 3 years about two medicine-related behaviors is considered important by the United States Pharmacopeia (Bush, 1999). They are what the child should do if he or she finds a pill on the floor or sees other kids getting into medicines. The answers, respectively, are "Give it to a grownup" and "Tell a grownup."

School-Age Children

When children reach the age of 5 or 6 years, they can be more actively involved when you educate them and their parents about their medicines. A good way to begin an interaction may be to ask the child about his or her favorite television show or hobby (Coulehan and Block, 1992). There can be a developmental range among elementary school children and great differences in their experiences with

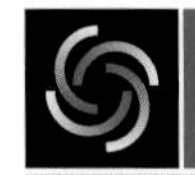

Box 11.3 What Children Want to Know About Medicines at Different Ages

CHILDREN IN KINDERGARTEN THROUGH FIRST GRADE

1. Why some medicines are only for children
2. How they can tell the difference between medicines for children and medicines for adults
3. The therapeutic purposes of medicines (e.g., prevention, cure, symptomatic relief)
4. Dose forms and ways of taking medicines
5. Importance of complying with the treatment regimen
6. The side effects of some medicines
7. If whether a medicine helps is related to its color, size, or taste

CHILDREN IN SECOND THROUGH FIFTH GRADE

1. What the ingredients are in medicines
2. How medicines work; where medicines go in the body
3. How doctors know that a medicine works
4. Why there are different medicines for different illnesses
5. Why the same medicine can be for different illnesses
6. Why there are different medicines for a single illness
7. Why you should not take other people's medicines

CHILDREN IN SIXTH THROUGH EIGHTH GRADE

1. Difference between prescription and OTC medicines
2. Meaning of dependency and addiction
3. How medicines are made
4. Why medicines come in different forms
5. Why one may have to adhere to a special diet and time schedule when taking a medicine
6. Potential for drug interactions with other medicines and foods
7. Lack of a relationship between the efficacy of a medicine and its source or price
8. Difference between brand and generic medicines
9. Difference between medicines, botanicals/herbs, and homeopathics
10. How to select an appropriate OTC medicine
11. For children born outside of the United States or whose parents are recent immigrants, differences between medicines produced in their country of origin and medicines produced elsewhere

medicines, which is why you need to ask children open-ended questions to assess their cognitive level and knowledge. Through simple questions such as "Why do you need to take this medicine?" or "How does the medicine work?" you can assess whether the child is starting to understand cause-and-effect relationships and that internal physiological mechanisms contribute to illness. If we consider Piaget's work, this typically happens around age 7, but it can happen when a child is somewhat younger or older.

Once a child begins to understand cause-and-effect relationships, you can give the child more details about how a medicine works in the body. You can also start to empower the child to begin to have some autonomy in medicine taking by saying "Work with your mom or dad in taking the medicine" instead of "Do not take the medicine unless your mom or dad is there." At this age, you also need to talk with the parent to ascertain how independent the child is becoming in medicine taking. Children with chronic conditions such as diabetes, epilepsy, or asthma may have a very good understanding of their disease and considerable autonomy in using them. For example, Sanz (2003) found that asthmatic children as young as 7 years old were able to give clear explanations about their disease and their medicines (how they worked, when they should be taken, and at which doses).

The information in Box 11.3 can be used by pharmacists who are invited into school classrooms to talk about their work and medicines. The recommended approach in this situation is to first engage the children in a conversation that will generate their questions. It has been found that taking some common medicines, pill boxes, inhalers, or other devices into the classroom stimulates children into talking about medicine use they have observed or have engaged in themselves and this leads to them asking questions about medicines (Menacker et al., 1999). The pharmacist-teacher can also engage the children in play-acting in which the children practice asking a pharmacist questions.

Adolescents

When children reach adolescence, you may want to spend part of the time communicating with the adolescent without the parents present. Pediatricians often ask parents to leave the room so they can communicate privately with adolescent children. Pharmacists can use the same technique. This allows you to build trust with the patient. Trust becomes especially important with adolescents. An adolescent may feel comfortable talking with you about birth control and sexually transmitted diseases if you sometimes talk with them independently of their parents. Adolescents need to know you will not tell their parents what they say or what they buy. You can typically give teenagers educational messages that would be the same as you would give an adult.

Summary

Communicating with and empowering children and parents to better understand their child's medical condition and medicine regimen can potentially improve patient adherence. Parents' beliefs about the seriousness of their child's medical condition or the severity of the complications their child might suffer if they do not take their medicines as prescribed relate positively to following recommended treatment regimens (DiMatteo, 2004). Also, parents may not understand what they have been told about their children's medicines by their physicians. For example, Riekert et al. (2003) found that even though physicians reported that a child was on a controller medicine for asthma, 38% of caregivers were not using a controller. You can assess the child's and parents' knowledge of the child's medical condition and medicine regimen and further educate them, as it is important for both parents and children to be appropriately educated about their medicines. Notably, in 2001, the International Pharmacy Federation supported such education by adopting a Statement of Principle, *The Pharmacist's Responsibility and Role in Teaching Children and Adolescents about Medicines*.

You need to use an empowering "patient-centered" interaction style when interacting with parents and children. Also, you need to remember to assess the cognitive developmental level of children through the use of open-ended questions. At the national level, the United States Pharmacopoeia has a position statement called "Ten Guiding Principles for Teaching Children and Adolescents about Medicines," which supports the right of children and adolescents to receive developmentally appropriate information and direct communications about medicines (Bush et al., 1999). Four of these ten guiding principles relate to pharmacist–parent–child communication. These four principles are an excellent summary of what you have learned in this chapter:

1. Children want to know. Health care providers and health educators should communicate directly with children about medicines.
2. Children's interest should be encouraged, and they should be taught how to ask questions of health care providers, parents, and other caregivers about medicines and other therapies.
3. Children, their parents, and their health care providers should negotiate the gradual transfer of responsibility for medicine use in ways that respect parental responsibilities and the health status and capabilities of the child.
4. Children's medicine education should take into account what children want to know about medicines, as well as what health care professionals think children should know.

REVIEW QUESTIONS

1. **Describe the "patient-centered" interaction style involved with medicine therapy for children and its relationship to empowerment.**
2. **What are the four stages of cognitive development proposed by Piaget?**
3. **What educational strategies would you use in each of Piaget's development stages?**
4. **Based on past research, what type of information should be the focus when educating a 7-year-old child about his or her medicines?**

REVIEW EXERCISE

After reading through the sample educational messages contained in Box 11.2, write down how the content of the message changed at each stage and how this reflects the cognitive level of the child. Next, pretend that you need to verbally educate a child at each stage of cognitive development about his or her diabetes medicines. Write down what you would say to a child at each level of development.

REFERENCES

Adams RJ, Smith BJ, Ruffin R. Impact of the physician's participatory style in asthma outcomes and patient satisfaction. *Annals of Allergy, Asthma & Immunology* 86:263–271, 2001.

Behrman RE, Vaughan VC III. *Textbook of Pediatrics*. Philadelphia, PA: WB Saunders, 1983.

Bush PJ (ed.). *Guide to Developing and Evaluating Medicine Education Programs and Materials for Children and Adolescents*. Rockville, MD: United States Pharmacopeial Convention, Inc., & American School Health Association, 1999.

Bush PJ, Davidson FR. Medicines and "drugs": What do children think? *Health Education Quarterly* 9:113–128, 1982.

Bush PJ, Hämeen-Anttila K. Children, adolescents, and medicines. In Rickles NM, Wertheimer AI, Smith MC (eds.). *Social and Behavioral Aspects of Pharmaceutical Care* (2nd ed., pp. 289–320). Boston, MA: Jones & Bartlett Press, 2009.

Bush PJ, Ozias JM, Walson PD, Ward RM. Ten guiding principles for teaching children and adolescents about medicines. *Clinical Therapeutics* 21:1280–1284, 1999.

Coulehan JL, Block MR. *The Medical Interview: A Primer for Students of the Art*. Philadelphia, PA: FA Davis, 1992.

DiMatteo MR. The role of effective communication with children and their families in fostering adherence to pediatric regimens. *Patient Education and Counseling* 55:339–344, 2004.

Hämeen-Anttila K, Juvonen M, Ahonen R, et al. What schoolchildren should be taught about medicines: Combined opinions of children and teachers. *Health Education* 105:424–436, 2005.

Iannotti RJ, Bush PJ. The development of autonomy in children's health behavior. In Sussman EJ, Feagans LV, Ray W (eds.). *Emotion, Cognition, Health, and Development in Children and Adolescents* (pp. 53–74). Hillsdale, NJ: Lawrence Erlbaum, 1992.

International Pharmaceutical Federation. FIP Statement of Principle: The pharmacist's responsibility and role in teaching children and adolescents about medicines, 2001 (www.fip.org). Accessed October 20, 2010.

Kelly GR, Scott JE. Medication compliance and health education among outpatients with chronic mental disorders. *Medical Care* 28:1181–1197, 1990.

Kieffer CH. Citizen empowerment: A developmental perspective. *Prevention in Human Services* 3:9–36,1984.

Lau RR, Klepper S. The development of illness orientations in children aged 6 through 12. *Journal of Health and Social Behavior* 29:149–168, 1988.

Menacker F, Aramburuzabala P, Minian N, et al. Children and medicines: What they want to know and how they want to learn. *Journal of Social and Administrative Pharmacy* 16:38–52, 1999.

O'Brien R, Bush P. Helping children learn how to use medicines. *Office Nurse* 6:14–19, 1993.

Piaget J. *The Moral Judgement of the Child*. New York: Harcourt, Brace, and World, Inc., 1932.

Ranelli P, Bartsch K, London K. Pharmacists' perceptions of children and families as medicine consumers. *Psychology and Health* 15:829–840, 2000.

Riekert KA, Butz AM, Eggleston PA, et al. Caregiver-physician medication concordance and undertreatment of asthma among inner-city children. *Pediatrics* 11:e214–e220, 2003.

Rodwell CM. An analysis of the concept of empowerment. *Journal of Advanced Nursing* 23:305–313, 1996.

Sanz EJ. Concordance and children's use of medicines. *British Medical Journal* 327:858–860, 2003.

Sleath B, Ayala GX, Davis S, et al. Child and caregiver-reported problems and concerns in using asthma medications. *Journal of Asthma* 47(6):633–638, 2010.

Sloand ED, Vessey JA. Self-medication with common household medicines by young adolescents. *Issues in Comprehensive Pediatric Nursing* 24:57–67, 2001.

Stewart M. Effective physician-patient communication and health outcomes: A review. *Canadian Medical Association Journal* 152:1423–1433, 1995.

Stewart M, Meredith L, Brown JB, Galajda J. The influence of older patient-physician communication on health and health-related outcomes. *Clinics in Geriatric Medicine* 16:25–36, 2000.

Street R, Piziak V, Carpentier W, et al. Provider-patient communication and metabolic control. *Diabetes Care* 16:714–721, 1993.

Tates K, Meeuwesen L. Doctor-parent-child communication. A review of the literature. *Social Science and Medicine* 52:839–851, 2001.

Wissow L, Roter D, Bauman LJ, et al. Patient-provider communication during the emergency department care of children with asthma. *Medical Care* 36:1439–1450, 1998.

CHAPTER

12

Interprofessional Collaboration and Effective Communication Skills

Overview

This chapter focuses on enhancing collaborative relationships between pharmacists and other health care providers in order to ensure better patient outcomes. The chapter first describes the value of establishing collaborative relationships as a means to improving patient care. The barriers and facilitators to developing these relationships are then described along with practical examples of effective strategies. The importance of building trust is highlighted, as well as the impact of using effective communication skills to strengthen trusting relationships. Finally, essential steps to building collaborative relationships are discussed. Many of these steps involve the same communication skills discussed in earlier chapters.

Pharmacist Roles in Collaborative Patient Care

The traditional process of prescribing a medication, dispensing a medication, monitoring a medication regimen, and adjusting medication therapy can be very disjointed, producing avoidable medication-related problems and contributing to poor health outcomes and significant increases in the cost of health care (Webb, 1995). Due to the significance of these medication-related problems, pharmacists are taking more active roles in the treatment of disease as well as the prevention of disease. According to Brushwood (2001), "Pharmacists have begun to assume new responsibilities that extend beyond ensuring accuracy and appropriateness in the processing of pharmaceutical orders—namely to assume the promotion of good therapeutic outcomes for patients." Thus, as responsible health care professionals, pharmacists realize they will be held accountable for the provision of appropriate patient care related to management of medication therapy. Many pharmacists are realizing they must work more closely with physicians and other health care providers to facilitate this process. The following practice research findings illustrate that it behooves pharmacists and other providers to engage in developing collaborative arrangements, knowing that:

- Research has found that pharmacists working in collaboration with physicians through a redesigned approach to medication use can prevent errors and reduce drug costs (Isetts et al., 2003).
- Patient adherence with medications significantly improves when pharmacists and physicians collaborate (Fredrick, 2003).
- Pharmacist–physician collaborative management of hypertension achieved consistent and significantly higher rates of blood pressure control compared to physician-only interventions (Weber et al., 2010).
- Confrontational relationships and procedural obstacles can be replaced with collaborative and trusting relationships when both physicians and pharmacists work on reducing feelings of discomfort about each other's skills, roles, and authority (Fredrick, 2003).

The collaborative movement has been most visible in the health care delivery reforms at the federal level. For example, pharmacist practitioners work closely with physicians to manage medication therapy within the Veterans Administration, Indian Health Service, and the Armed Services health care systems. Reform at the state level is evidenced by numerous changes to the pharmacy scope of practice laws. For example, many state laws and regulations have added to their definition of the practice of pharmacy such wording as "Pharmacists have the responsibility for initiating, modifying, or discontinuing drug therapy in accordance with written protocols or agreements established and approved by a practitioner authorized to prescribe such drugs."

This approach of redefining the scope of pharmacy practice has garnered a great deal of public support. In fact, most states and the federal government have enacted legislation allowing for some form of collaborative practice for pharmacists. Due to this legislative and regulatory reform, pharmacists are now empowered to participate in a more active way in patient care with physicians and other prescribers. Within these legislative initiatives, pharmacists are not asking for the privilege of independent prescribing since they realize they have very limited training in the diagnostic skills expected of physicians. Most collaborative legislation requires written protocols between a prescriber and a pharmacist. In addition, physicians must voluntarily enter into these agreements in which both parties take joint responsibility for the oversight and outcomes of medication therapy management. Thus, as will be discussed later in further detail, a key element for the implementation of these collaborative partnerships is a strong feeling of trust and confidence among participants.

Other examples of successful collaborative relationships appear in the medication therapy management or MTM programs that are emerging in a variety of patient care settings. MTM programs are distinct services or groups of services that optimize therapeutic outcomes for individual patients (APhA, 2008). They attempt to maximize therapeutic outcomes and reduce the risk of adverse events, including adverse drug reactions, by ensuring more appropriate medication use. Core elements of MTM services include medication therapy reviews, personal medication records, medication action plans, interventions and/or referrals, and documentation and follow-up. These core elements focus on creating solutions for patient-specific medication therapy problems and collaborating with other health care professionals. Effective MTM programs require solid collaborative relationships between pharmacists and other health care providers. Such collaborations require pharmacists to share responsibility for medication therapy outcomes and give them opportunities to apply their clinical training and skills. Studies have shown that pharmacist-led MTM programs have proven to be valuable, showing improvements in clinical, economic, and humanistic outcomes (Bunting et al., 2008; Fera et al., 2008). The expanding roles for pharmacists within patient care programs, such as MTM, are reinforcing a public perception that pharmacists are among the most reliable, trusted, and accessible health care providers (Tindall and Millonig, 2003).

Barriers and Facilitators to Collaborative Partnerships

A growing body of health care literature is championing the development of interdisciplinary collaborations as the best way to provide health services. These strategies are especially needed to treat patients with complex therapies who require multiple sets of services or who need both acute and chronic care services. While the wisdom for such collaboration is well documented, and several successful practices exist, the practice is not as widespread as desired. It is interesting to note that such collaborations existed in previous decades as "small-town doctors" and "corner druggists" worked together. However, these collaborations were eroded by several factors, including the rise of managed care and the depersonalization of relationships between patients and health care providers that have strained the patient–provider relationship. In order to better understand the current emergence of more collaborative relationships, an analysis of the perceived barriers and facilitators to collaborative practice is warranted.

POTENTIAL BARRIERS

In many situations, expansion of collaborative practices is inhibited by the attitudes of some providers that indicate reservations about giving pharmacists a

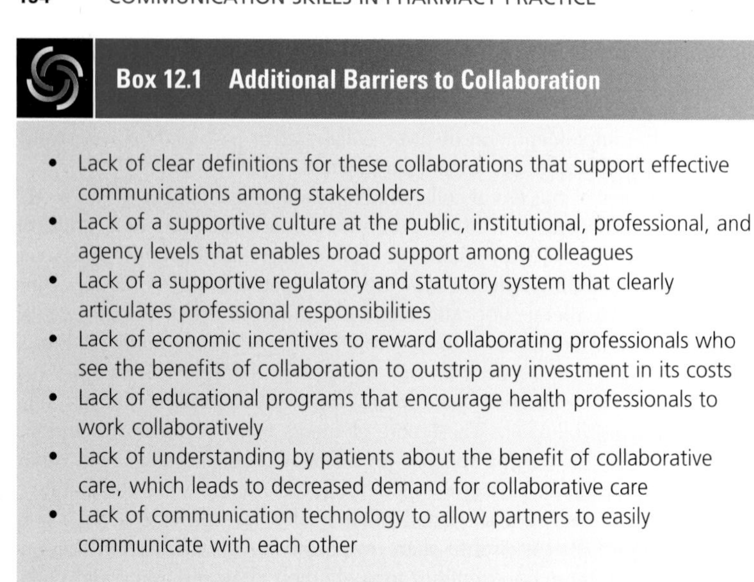

Box 12.1 Additional Barriers to Collaboration

- Lack of clear definitions for these collaborations that support effective communications among stakeholders
- Lack of a supportive culture at the public, institutional, professional, and agency levels that enables broad support among colleagues
- Lack of a supportive regulatory and statutory system that clearly articulates professional responsibilities
- Lack of economic incentives to reward collaborating professionals who see the benefits of collaboration to outstrip any investment in its costs
- Lack of educational programs that encourage health professionals to work collaboratively
- Lack of understanding by patients about the benefit of collaborative care, which leads to decreased demand for collaborative care
- Lack of communication technology to allow partners to easily communicate with each other

greater role in drug therapy decision making (Alkhateeb et al., 2009). As pharmacists seek to expand their roles and attempt to develop collaborative practice arrangements, they will have to overcome the perception by some physicians that increased pharmacist activity in patient care is an encroachment on their professional territory. However, recent successes (especially in institutional settings and within special populations such as geriatrics) should resolve some of these issues. Additional barriers to collaboration appear in Box 12.1.

POTENTIAL FACILITATORS

Fortunately, many activities in today's health care environment involve health professionals working together in teams. The most successful collaborations appear to involve health care providers who share the same discipline (infectious diseases, geriatrics, or pediatrics). Collaboration within disciplines is facilitated by common perceptions, language, values, and interdisciplinary socialization. Such collaborations provide evidence that when people find ways to work together, there is an increase in productivity and innovation (Conference Board of Canada, 2005). When collaborations are successful, synergy occurs, and the output of the whole is much larger than the sum of the individuals involved (see Box 12.2). The old wise axiom that two heads are better than one holds true when it comes to strengthening relationships between pharmacists and other health care providers. That means both can see the wisdom of trying to achieve something via comprehensive, patient-centered partnerships that neither professional could achieve alone. When both see the wisdom of these collaborative partnerships, they will work toward finding the most appropriate structure to organize, plan, and implement their collaborative

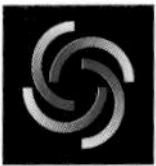

Box 12.2 Four Key Characteristics of Effective Collaboration

1. **Sharing:** Includes sharing of responsibilities, philosophies of health care, values, planning, interventions, and perspectives such as commitment to patient-centered care
2. **Partnering:** Implies that two or more people will join together in a collegial, authentic, and productive relationship characterized by honest communication, mutual trust, and respect. In addition, partners value the work and perspectives of the other professionals in the partnership, and each works toward common goals having specific outcomes.
3. **Interdependency:** Refers to the fact that professionals are interdependent, rather than autonomous, as they work toward meeting patient needs.
4. **Power:** Seen as being shared among partners with empowerment accorded to all participants, including patients. Sharing of power is based on knowledge and experience rather than functions or titles (University of Toronto, 2004).

efforts. Recent experience has shown that patient care is improved when pharmacists and other providers engage in building collaborative partnerships using the following strategies:

- Recognize they are creating opportunities for change as like-minded individuals come together to tackle an issue important to their common patients
- Mobilize resources to create change
- Develop a shared vision of what long-term change will be as they strive for better health outcomes that transcend personal interests
- Seek involvement of other diverse and nontraditional partners
- Choose an effective group structure to assist with open, honest, and trusting communication
- Develop some type of feedback system so lessons learned can be shared with others

Although developing collaborative relationships takes time and attention to detail, there are many catalysts to initiate these partnerships. Typically, individual practitioners or groups of practitioners can stimulate change at the local level by realizing that two or more professionals need to work together to meet patient needs. Following this recognition, a pilot project may be initiated to build potential strategies addressing the need and to build trust among the individuals involved. If successful on a small scale, the team may then decide to expand the collaboration to tackle larger issues or expand efforts to a wider audience. Positive experiences may spark additional interest in collaboration by other health care providers. Most collaborative partnerships eventually evolve into more formalized arrangements where parties:

- Share a common understanding of the context of their collaboration
- Identify the collaboration partners
- Develop mechanisms to govern themselves
- Develop mechanisms to handle shared revenues and expenses
- Advocate for any needed legislation or professional standards that would strengthen their partnership and stimulate other partnerships
- Develop guidelines for partner relationships
- Clearly define their target community
- Determine how varying professional cultural issues are handled
- Establish criteria for when the collaboration may be dissolved in the future

Initial Steps to Developing Collaborative Arrangements

The following sections focus on developing collaborative relationships with physicians. However, many of the same strategies can be used to develop partnerships with other health care providers, such as nurse practitioners, physician assistants, dietitians, physical therapists, and others. It would be redundant to apply all these strategies to every conceivable partner. Thus, the authors have chosen to illustrate these approaches using physicians as the partnering group. Additional strategies are also listed in Box 12.3.

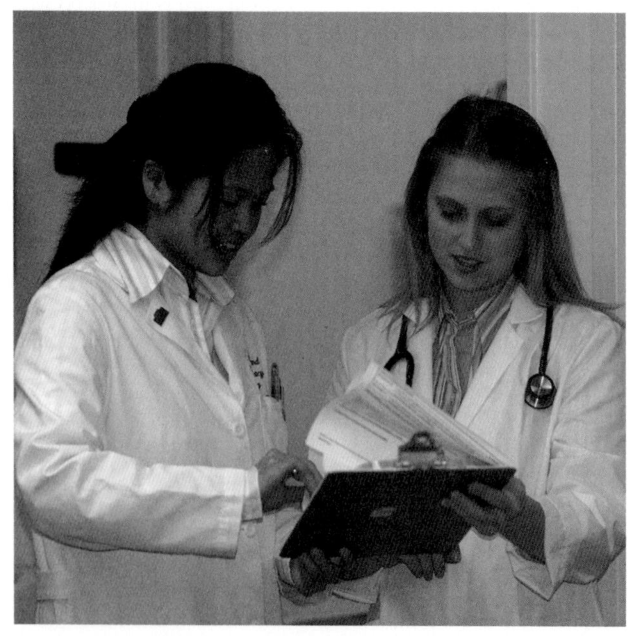

Pharmacist and physician discussing patient's laboratory results.

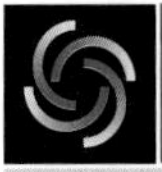

Box 12.3 Strategies to Build Collaborative Relationships

1. Develop joint statements that support patient rights to be involved in making informed decisions affecting drug therapy and that articulate the value that patient trust, safety, and relationships with caregivers always come first.
2. Host jointly sponsored professional meetings, especially at the local level, to help develop widespread understanding and awareness of physician and pharmacist responsibilities in drug therapy and why collaborative approaches to drug therapy benefit all.
3. Build effective communication, administrative, and documentation systems that allow pharmacists to share relevant patient information in accordance with applicable ethical standards, accepted medical and pharmacy practices, and state/federal statutes and regulations to provide continuity of care for patients.
4. Stimulate the development of technology to enhance communication within collaborative practices (e.g., shared patient databases relevant to drug therapy).
5. Volunteer to work jointly on committees and projects that enhance patient education and adherence, investigate drug therapy issues, and promote better practice guidelines.
6. Start with a project that has a limited scope, such as monitoring patients on warfarin or patients with diabetes. Expand services after documenting impact.

Before you embark on any collaborative practice, you should be able to answer three key questions, the first being "*What local conditions support or inhibit any attempt at making a collaborative effort?*" Learning about a community's readiness for expanded pharmacists' roles begins with talking with key stakeholders, such as patients, hospitals, third-party administrators, and local and state physician groups, which may be influenced by your collaborative efforts. Hopefully, these contacts will provide you with important insights and understanding about the viability of these collaborative relationships. For example, strong advocates for comprehensive medication therapy management may be patient or community groups about to receive this care. Getting them on your "bandwagon" is a great strategy to gather support while developing initial relationships with physicians. When the time comes to approach physicians, it will be much easier if you have done your homework and have identified the following:

- Health care practitioners who have an interest in the proposed partnership
- Patients or patient groups (broad-based and influential) who may benefit from your partnership

- Individuals willing to share time and resources to make your collaboration work
- Community agencies and media interests who would like to see your collaboration succeed and contribute to your community and are willing to support your effort
- Examples of other collaborative relationships that have worked with descriptions of their structure and governance

Secondly, when interacting with physicians, you should ask yourself: "*Am I using the physician's limited time efficiently and wisely?*" Practice your verbal presentation before your meeting since the first few moments of your interaction will be critical to the physicians' overall impression of you and your ideas. In addition, review your written materials to make sure they reinforce your verbal communication to articulate your ideas and concerns. Try to avoid using technical jargon so as to facilitate reaching a common understanding of what is being presented. Speak in terms they can understand and appreciate, especially if you have to be specific about state practice acts or other complex subjects.

Finally you should ask: "*Have I assured myself that I have the trust of the physician that I am hoping to work with?*" In addition to refining your verbal and written message, you must also acknowledge the value of establishing trust as you start to develop collaborative relationships. Effective collaborative relationships begin with mutual trust or a "shared belief that you can depend on each other to achieve a common purpose" or "having faith in the integrity, consistency, and commitment of each other" (Gillies, 2001).

Building Trust: The Cornerstone to Successful Collaborative Arrangements

In studying successful collaborative practices, Zillich (2004) found that the majority of the 340 primary care physicians he interviewed reported that the most influential driver in their relationship with pharmacists was trustworthiness. Another study (Howard and Trim, 2003) reported that the development of a trusting relationship was important in collaborations between physicians and the expanded role of pharmacists. Tallia et al. (2003) explored this important factor and also found the number one contributing element to the success of collaborative partnerships was the strength of their trusting relationships. The specific behaviors in those trusting relationships were that both parties:

- Sought input from one another
- Allowed each other to do their jobs without unnecessary oversight
- Openly discussed success and failure and learned from both

While there is a widespread consensus on the importance of having trust, there is little consensus on how to define it (Mayer et al., 1995). To some, having trust in others relates to predictable behavior. For our purposes, this would mean that physicians would be able to assess the probability of how pharmacists would act in a certain way. For example, if physicians have had bad experiences or even no experiences with pharmacists, they may feel that, although well intended, pharmacists do not have the skills to contribute to collaborative relationships in a meaningful way. However, if physicians are confident in pharmacists' past behavior and can predict a successful outcome, they will have greater trust in pharmacists and believe they will not have to "watch the pharmacist's each and every action." Trust between physicians and pharmacists cannot be decreed or legislated. The willingness of physicians to work with pharmacists is a combination of shared values, attitudes, and interests. Trust is built by the confidence one has in another person's predictable behavior or the security one has in a person's representations. Factors that influence the development of trust include the following:

- Consistent behavior over time reinforces positive or negative feelings about trust.
- Common goals or vision help strengthen trusting relationships.
- Mutual respect for each other should exist.
- How the individual parties react when the relationship is strained (e.g., when a medication error occurs) could weaken or strengthen the relationship.
- Mutual understanding of any economic gain from the partnership.

Using Communication Skills to Enhance Collaborative Relationships

The success of our collaborations with physicians depends on effective communication skills since pharmacists and physicians come from two diverse professional cultures. Both parties must have the ability to articulate their perceptions and knowledge in an understandable manner and to use effective listening skills to gain an understanding of the meaning and context of each other's messages. They must be willing to receive feedback from each other, as discussed in earlier chapters. An awareness of the other person's perceptions is critical to developing strong trusting relationships. Perceptions that appear to be essential to forming collaborative interactions include the following:

- Does this person share in my goals?
- Does this individual recognize that we are creating opportunities for change as like-minded individuals to tackle an issue important to our patients?
- Does this person have the required knowledge and ability to help us reach our goals?
- Will this person stick to his or her commitments and be reliable?
- Will this person share with me information that I need to know?
- Does this person want me to be successful as a partner in this intervention?
- Is what we are doing creating real value that will be of service to patients?

Trust will grow between collaborators when both perceive a high degree of predictability of one another's behavior. In addition, trust occurs when individuals perceive that the other party will not engage in opportunistic behavior that exploits a position of power or the vulnerabilities of another. Communication that emanates from strong collaborations should portray each of its players as equals.

For example, public communications about a collaborative medication therapy management program should position the patient as the beneficiary so that physicians and pharmacists are seen as collaborating on the patient's behalf. Otherwise the public might perceive this activity as benefiting either the pharmacist or the physician at the expense of the other party.

Five Critical Behaviors Within Collaborative Partnerships

1. **Relationships have long-term and short-term agendas.** Pharmacist–physician partnerships should have long-term and short-term agendas, as there are often struggles between the desire to take immediate action and the need to plan for a sustained effort. There are no specific formulas for how much time and energy to allocate for building relationships or for planning strategies. However, experienced partnerships agree that both activities are essential to long-term success.
2. **Relationships are nonhierarchical and based on equality.** In a true interprofessional collaboration, partners relate to each other on a nonhierarchical basis, regardless of their position in the organizational structure of the practice. No single organization or individual should dominate or control the decision-making process. Goals for the collaboration should be set that are broader than the goals of any participating organization or individual and that cannot be reached through the efforts of any single group. Since equality in the relationship is essential in collaborations, participants should believe their input is valued and they are making a meaningful contribution. Working in these types of relationships may be difficult for some physicians who have been trained in hierarchical, competitive, top-down structures. They may be used to achieving their goals only with other physicians and may not value collaboration with nonphysicians since they must share power, knowledge, and influence (Lieberman and Grolnick, 1997). It may also be difficult for some pharmacists who don't want too much "responsibility" and have been trained simply to dispense products.
3. **Collaborations should consider patient perspectives.** Patients bring unique perspectives and opportunities to strengthen physician–pharmacist partnerships. Many patients are used to working with teams of health care providers and many perceive the value of such collaborations. Patients may even demand that their care providers work as organized teams. Patients may also be more knowledgeable about their community's culture and the local health care network. They may help identify perceived leaders in the health care environment and who might facilitate or block progress in developing collaborative relationships. Thus, pharmacists should utilize patient knowledge and perceptions of the community and health care environment when developing collaborative relationships.
4. **Trust and shared visions are central to these relationships.** Diversity among partners adds strength to the collaboration. However, such diversity may also be a source of concern if common values and visions are not shared.

An effective strategy for shaping a group of diverse individuals is to concentrate on common ground (i.e., helping people get the best use of their medicine, reducing polypharmacy in a geriatric population, reducing preventable errors in medication taking) and to develop a unified vision for what will constitute success (i.e., reducing major hospital admissions due to medication errors by 50% in 1 year). In addition, if a particular group of physicians or pharmacists has not worked together in the past, they must trust each other on an interpersonal level even though they may not know each other. Once people have familiarized themselves with each other, it becomes easier to identify areas of common interest. As physicians and pharmacists explore perspectives and find common ground, they can begin to shape a vision that will guide them into stronger collaborative practice arrangements. This shaping process typically progresses from initial discussions, to a consensus agreement, and then to a final written vision statement that reflects the conditions, interests, and issues of the partnering professionals. It is wise to take the time to let this process unfold to allow buy-in from all parties.

5. **Relationships should demonstrate respect for each profession's culture.** Collaborative practice arrangements are best when those within the collaboration recognize, understand, and value the culture of each other's profession. Relationships weaken when one of the partners believes there is little respect for his/her culture or skill.

Collaboration and the Patient-Centered Medical Home

One emerging approach to providing patient care that requires strong collaborative relationships is the patient-centered medical home. The Patient Protection and Affordable Care Act (PPACA) of 2010 contains provisions designed to enhance the coordination and quality of primary health care in the country (HR 3590, Public Law 111-148). Provisions in the PPACA provide grants to develop community-based collaborative care networks and increase Medicare reimbursements for primary care services.

One of the provisions also promotes development of "health homes" (also known as medical homes), which are primary care sites that qualify for enhanced reimbursement for coordinating care for Medicaid patients with chronic diseases. To qualify as a medical home, the primary care site must assure comprehensive, coordinated care among multiple providers, in part through the use of information technology to integrate care. The medical home concept is designed to enhance continuity of care by promoting an integrated team approach to the provision of primary care, especially the treatment of chronic disease. It rewards preventive care and establishes partnerships among providers, patients, and families. The active involvement of pharmacists has been identified as crucial to the success of medical homes (Smith et al., 2010). Key to the success of this new approach will be effective communication between health care providers themselves and between team members and patients. Thus, as health care providers establish these primary care sites, they must develop strong communication processes between health care providers and effective communication linkages between providers and patients.

Summary

Collaborations between health professionals are promising modes of professional behavior that will address many of the pressing needs of 21st century health care. Collaborative practices are more than just passing fads. There is a growing realization that in order to provide effective and comprehensive health care, health care professionals must collaborate with each other, with each profession bringing different areas of competence to assure better patient care. Collaboration with other health professionals, especially between physicians and pharmacists, provides additional opportunities for professional growth and fulfillment for both parties. Professionals who participate in these collaborative relationships combine their independent skill sets in a commitment to share power, resources, and problem-solving talent for the betterment of someone other than themselves. The cornerstone of what makes all this work is shared trust and confidence in each other.

Effective collaborations occurring between two people who represent the same or different disciplines are characterized by:

- The coordination of individual actions
- Cooperation in planning and working together
- Sharing of goals, planning, and problem solving
- Sharing of decision making and responsibility

The issues within collaborative practice and comprehensive medication therapy management do not just involve revamping statutory definitions or regulations of what constitutes the medical and pharmacy practice. They also involve pharmacists and physicians continually revisiting their relationships as they work to meet the continuously expanding health care needs of patients and families.

REVIEW QUESTIONS

1. **What are three barriers to interprofessional collaboration that exist in institutional practice? Community-based practice?**
2. **What are four characteristics of effective collaborative relationships?**
3. **State three strategies to develop trust between pharmacists and other health care providers.**
4. **How do you develop a shared vision with other health care providers?**

REVIEW CASE

REVIEW CASE STUDY 12.1

Mary Simpson is a 25-year-old recent PharmD graduate who is a staff pharmacist for a mid-sized chain of pharmacies. She recently attended a workshop on collaborative medication therapy management and decided to approach a group of nearby family medicine physicians. Convinced she has something to offer these physicians, she schedules a visit at their offices on a Wednesday morning. Mary visits Victor Diaz, a seasoned physician with 20 years of practice, and states, "I believe if we work together, I can help you see a difference in the therapeutic outcomes of your elderly patients..." Mary explains the various elements of collaborative MTM and continues, "All I need from you is your permission to let me start a collaborative MTM program as allowed by our state practice laws."

Dr. Diaz says, "Uh! OK! Well, we'll see, but since you're here, what can you recommend for an 83-year-old lady who is very much riddled with anxiety? I am thinking of a benzodiazepine. What do you think?"

Mary seizes this opening to discuss this with Dr. Diaz and remembers the general rule to "start low and go slow" when dosing elderly people. After their discussion, Dr. Diaz says, "I really must get back to work, but I will discuss your idea with our group and we will get back to you in a week." Mary returns to her pharmacy feeling that their meeting went very well.

A month goes by and she has not heard from Dr. Diaz, nor has he returned her follow-up phone calls. Somewhat discouraged, Mary tells her story to Fred Miller, a 55-year-old pharmacist who shares a shift with her. After hearing Mary's story, Fred comments, "Well, I am not surprised, they are a pretty closed group." Fred goes on to ask Mary a few questions: "Mary, what makes you think Dr. Diaz and his group would welcome you as a collaborative colleague? What 'homework' have you done to present facts and figures to Dr. Diaz about the need for what you are trying to accomplish? What have you done in the past 6 months to establish his trust and confidence? Now that you have opened this door, what are you going to do to make this happen?"

During the following week, Mary considers Fred's questions, weighing possible responses, and then says to Fred, "I need your advice again. Help me write a plan to present to Dr. Diaz and his colleagues. I need to make him understand what I am talking about. Fred, can you help me do this?"

As you consider the material presented in this chapter, what further advice you would give Mary if you were Fred so that she would better understand how to establish a collaborative partnership?

REFERENCES

Alkhateeb FM, Unni E, Latif D, et al. Physician attitudes toward collaborative agreements with pharmacists and their expectations of community pharmacists' responsibilities in West Virginia. *Journal of the American Pharmaceutical Association* 49(6):797–800, 2009.

American Pharmacists Association and National Association of Chain Drug Stores Foundation. Medication therapy management in community pharmacy practice: Core elements of an MTM service. *Journal of the American Pharmaceutical Association* 48 (3):341–353, 2008.

Bunting BA, Smith BH, Sutherland SE. The Asheville Project: Clinical and economic outcomes of a community-based long-term medication therapy management program for hypertension and dyslipidemia. *Journal of the American Pharmaceutical Association* 48 (1):23–31, 2008.

Brushwood DB. From confrontation to collaboration: Collegial accountability and the expanding role of pharmacists in the management of chronic pain. *The Journal of Law, Medicine and Ethics* 29:69–93, 2001.

Conference Board of Canada. *The Enhancing Interdisciplinary Collaboration in Primary Health*. Toronto, 2005.

Fera T, Bluml BM, Ellis WM, et al. The Diabetes Ten City Challenge: Interim clinical and humanistic outcomes of a multistate community pharmacy diabetes care program. *J Am Pharm Assoc* 48 (2):181–190, 2008.

Fredrick J. Patient compliance increases with collaboration. *Drug Store News* 8:12, 2003.

Gillies RR. Physician-system relationships: Stumbling blocks and promising practices. *Medical Care* 39(Suppl 1):105–106, 2001.

Howard M, Trim K. Collaboration between community pharmacists and family physicians: Lessons learned from the seniors medication assessment research trial. *Journal of the American Medical Association* 43:566–572, 2003.

Isetts BJ, Brown LM, Schondelmeyer SW, et al. Quality assessment of a collaborative approach for decreasing drug-related morbidity and achieving therapeutic goals. *Archives of Internal Medicine* 163:1813–1820, 2003.

Lieberman A, Grolnick M. Networks, reform, and the professional development of teachers. In Hargreaves A (ed.). *Rethinking Educational Change with Heart and Mind* (p. 207). Alexandria, VA: Association for Supervision and Curriculum Development, 1997.

Mayer RC, Davis JH, Schoorman FD. In integrative model of organizational trust. *The Academy of Management Review* 20:709–734, 1995.

Smith M, Bates DW, Bodenheimer T, Cleary PD. Why pharmacists belong in the medical home. *Health Affairs* 29:906–913, 2010.

Tallia AF, Stange KC, McDonald RR. Understanding organizational design of primary care practice. *Journal of Healthcare Management* 48:45–59, 2003.

Tindall WN, Millonig MK. *Pharmaceutical Care: Insights from Community Pharmacists*. Boca Rotan, FL: CRC Press, 2003.

Webb EC. Prescribing medication: Changing the paradigm for a changing healthcare system. *American Journal of Health-System Pharmacy* 52:1693–1695, 1995.

Weber CA, Ernst ME, Sezate GS, et al. Pharmacist-physician comanagement of hypertension and reduction in 24-hour ambulatory blood pressures. *Archives of Internal Medicine* 170(18):1634–1639, 2010.

Zillich AJ, McDonough RP, Carter BL, et al. Influential characteristics of physician/pharmacist collaborative relationships. *Annals of Pharmacotherapy* 38:764–770, 2004.

RECOMMENDED READINGS

Institute of Medicine. Committee on Quality of Health Care in America. *Crossing the Quality Chasm: A New Health System for the 21st Century*. Washington, DC: National Academy Press, 2001.

Lindeke LL, Block DE. Interdisciplinary collaboration in the 21st century. *Minnesota Medicine* 84:1–6, 2001.

Pew Health Professions Commission. *Critical Challenges: Revitalizing the Health Professions for the 21st Century*. San Francisco, CA: UCSF Center for the Health Professions, 1995.

University of Toronto. *Interdisciplinary Education for Collaborative Patient-centered Practice* (p. 66). Ottawa: Health Canada, 2004.

Zellmer W. Collaborative drug therapy management. *American Journal of Health-System Pharmacy* 52:1732, 1995.

CHAPTER

13

Electronic Communication in Health Care

JEFF J. CAIN, KEVIN A. CLAUSON, AND BRENT I. FOX

Overview

Health care professionals have been using electronic media for several years to communicate with patients and amongst themselves. Although e-mail and the Internet are common tools used by both health care providers and patients, recent developments pertaining to social media and mobile applications have created new opportunities and novel challenges.

The possibilities and issues associated with electronic communications are numerous and often very complex. This chapter examines the use of digital media for health care communications, including traditional (e.g., e-mail) and contemporary (e.g., social media) forms. In addition, special attention will be given to current technology trends that may point to future possibilities and issues.

Introduction

While this chapter attempts to address the current use of digital media for health care communications, the technologies evolve so rapidly that newer forms will continue to supplement or even supplant the examples cited. However, many of the overarching issues will remain, regardless of the medium or application. Patient privacy, communication efficiencies, legal considerations, and other issues continue to be important topics even though the technology landscape continues to shift at a remarkable pace. In examining these issues, this chapter will:

- Provide the background information necessary to comprehend the current use of the Internet for health care
- Describe issues and opportunities pertaining to electronic communications in patient–provider relationships
- Describe issues and opportunities pertaining to electronic communications in interprofessional relationships
- Describe issues and opportunities for using social media in health care
- Describe legal issues pertaining to electronic communications in health care
- Identify and discuss trends in communications
- Describe guidelines for using e-mail and social media in health care communications

Foundations of Internet-Based Communication

HISTORICAL PERSPECTIVES

We could spend considerable time and pages discussing the complete history of the Internet. However, we will focus on a small set of important milestones and encourage interested readers to explore the information found in the chapter references. The Internet's origins date back more than 40 years to research conducted at the Defense Advanced Research Project Agency (DARPA). The Advanced Research Projects Agency Network (ARPANET) grew out of DARPA's work and was focused on developing a global computer communications infrastructure. Throughout the 1970s, ARPANET was primarily the sandbox for researchers and government agencies, with a focus on military and defense uses (Fox, 2005; Heussner, 2009; Leiner et al., 2010).

Those who follow the information technology industry have likely observed that most technological innovations follow a common pattern, where widespread adoption of the technology by the public often follows the development of what is commonly called the "killer app." Killer apps are the software applications whose popularity is so strong that it guarantees success of the technology on which it runs (Merriam-Webster, 2011). The first network e-mail message, sent in 1972, just a few years after ARPANET was developed, became the killer app for what was to become today's Internet. Ironically, the network e-mail function was developed out of a need for ARPANET researchers to communicate, not for the general public to communicate (Leiner et al., 2011).

Advancements in the early 1990s truly opened the Internet to the common public. Sir Tim Berners-Lee and colleagues at CERN (European Organization for Nuclear Research) publicly introduced the World Wide Web in 1991 (Ward, 2006). Web browser applications like Mosaic began appearing a few years later, and public interest in and use of the Internet exploded. Like others, you may interchangeably use "Web" and "Internet" to describe your online experience. In reality, the Internet is the underlying network on which the Web operates, allowing anyone to navigate online without the technical expertise needed prior to the invention of the Web (Lee, 2004).

As more people began using the Web, e-mail became immensely popular. The source of e-mail's popularity is easily identified: It allows global communication that is free and almost instantaneous. According to data from May 2010, 78% of adult Americans use the Internet on an average day, and 94% of adult Internet users use e-mail (Pew Internet, 2010). Box 13.1 lists other popular activities of adult Internet users.

E-MAIL COMMUNICATION

There are clear implications for pharmacists from the data presented in Box 13.1. E-mail remains the killer app for the Internet in the United States. The continued popularity of e-mail is beginning to permeate how people manage their health, where you now see patients desiring to communicate with their providers using e-mail or secure messaging systems that are similar in concept and function (Liederman and Morefield, 2003; Sittig et al., 2001; Fashner and Drye, 2011). There are several considerations for any health care provider who wants to communicate with patients via e-mail.

Box 13.1 Sample Activities Performed by U.S. Adult Internet Users

Internet Activity	Internet Users (%)
E-mail	94
Use a search engine	87
Look for medical information	83
Get news	75
Go online for fun	72
Buy a product	72
Visit a video-sharing site	66
Use a social networking site	61
Send instant messages	47
Share photos	46
Read someone else's blog	32
Use status-update service	17

The first consideration is privacy and security of the message. E-mail communication is subject to provisions of the Health Insurance Portability and Accountability Act (HIPAA), so caution and diligence are necessary to ensure that protected health information (PHI) is not shared in a manner that allows anyone other than patients (or their caregivers) to access the message. Recent methods to address this concern utilize a model in which providers and patients create messages in a secure online location, often known as a portal. The intended recipients then receive an e-mail notification to log into the secure portal to read/act on the message. The advantage of this model is that the information is never actually transmitted via e-mail. Instead, it is housed in a secure online environment (Lin et al., 2005).

In addition to portals, traditional e-mail systems have been used to communicate with patients. In a pharmacy, one of the more common uses of traditional e-mail is to notify a patient that a prescription is ready for pickup, usually simply indicating that "a prescription is ready" or that "prescription number X is ready." These messages do not risk exposing PHI because nothing specific to the patient is included.

The second consideration regarding patient–provider e-mail communication is reimbursement. Today's health care system is facing a staggering number of patients, creating extreme pressure on providers to deliver care for so many people. The reality is that providers must be reimbursed for the services they provide—including e-mail communication—to maintain their practice. A relatively small number of private insurers are reimbursing for e-mail communication (Freudenheim, 2005), and currently it is not widespread enough to encourage physicians to adopt it fully in practice. Using e-mail for practice will likely not gain widespread acceptance until Medicare begins reimbursing, even though patients' desire for and satisfaction with this service is growing (Stalberg et al., 2008; Lightspeed Research, 2009; Fashner and Drye, 2011). The future of pharmacist reimbursement for e-mail communication is unknown, but it will likely not occur before physician reimbursement is widespread.

Community pharmacy practitioners can likely predict the third challenge of e-mail communication: changes in workflow. The introduction of a new communication method into a complex system can lead to problems such as confusion, distraction, and frustration due to unclear expectations. The first point that patients must understand is that e-mail communication should never be used for urgent needs. Patients must understand that e-mail is best used for appointment scheduling, requesting a refill, obtaining test results, clarifying billing questions, and similar topics. Patients should also be given a general time frame for how fast their e-mails will be addressed and what topics are appropriate for e-mail communication. On the provider side, policies should be established and communicated regarding who is responsible for e-mail communication, just as policies exist for handling phone calls. Policies should also delineate who is responsible for ensuring that e-mail communication becomes part of the patient's record.

These challenges represent the primary impediments to patient–provider e-mail exchange becoming commonplace. While the challenges may seem daunting, they are but another evolutionary change our health care system will undergo as a result of the dynamic nature of technology and cultural changes in our country.

THE INTERNET AS A SOURCE OF INFORMATION

Referring back to Box 13.1, you can see that Americans continue to value the Internet as a source of medical information. In fact, since the early 2000s, Americans have turned to the Internet to find medical information. Looking closely, Internet users seek information about specific diseases and treatments. They also search for information on doctors and other providers as seen in Box 13.2 (Fox, 2011). While these uses of the Internet are not explicit examples of Internet-based *communication*, the sustained popularity of the Internet for locating medical information warrants your thoughts. A decade's worth of data indicate that patients value the Internet as an information source. As an extension of that importance, patients take action based on the information they find online, often seeking additional guidance and treatment from qualified providers. In terms of pharmacists' practice, patients do now and will continue to show up or call the pharmacy (and, in the future, send text messages) with questions based on the information they find online.

SOCIAL USES OF THE INTERNET

Another emerging trend that pharmacists are seeing in their practice is the popularity of interactive social uses of the Internet. These uses represent a relatively

Box 13.2 Popular Health-Related Topics of Adult U.S. Internet Users

Health-Related Topics	Internet Users (%)
Specific disease/problem information	66
Specific treatment/procedure information	56
Doctor or other health professional	44
Hospitals or other medical facilities	36
Health insurance	33
Food safety or recalls	29
Drug safety or recalls	24
Environmental hazards	22

Source: Fox S. *Health topics*. February 2, 2011. Retrieved February 25, 2011 from http://pewinternet.org/reports/2011/healthtopics.aspx.

recent development in American society and are beginning to rival traditional uses of the Internet, such as making purchases (as seen in Box 13.1). We expand considerably on this topic below; however, here you are encouraged to think about both your personal and professional social uses of the Internet:

- Do you connect with friends and family members through online services such as Facebook, Plaxo, or LinkedIn?
- Have any patients sent you a "friend" request on Facebook?
- Are you a member of a pharmacy-specific social networking site?
- Are you actively updating colleagues about your professional experiences using an updating service like Twitter?
- Have any patients asked you to let them know their prescriptions are ready for pickup via Twitter?
- Have you identified a core group of blogs that you follow because the authors post intriguing comments?
- Is your pharmacy using YouTube to provide information to its patients?

These questions represent a small sample of the growing number of social uses of the Internet in today's health care environment. In thinking about your answers and your own social uses of the Internet, it is easy to identify why this form of Internet-based communication is popular. Eysenbach (2008) identified five core features of social uses of the Internet for health-related activities that apply to our discussion:

- Social networking: the building of relationships or connections among people
- Participation: the direct involvement of patients in the management of their own health care and health-related information
- Apomediation: the identification of trustworthy health-related information and services through the use of a collaborative filtering process
- Collaboration: the connecting of people who would not normally be able to connect
- Openness: the ability to move patient information across separate systems

These characteristics are enabling the growth of the Internet as a social communications tool. This growth will impact pharmacy practice, and you should consider these characteristics as you read about the topics below.

CONSIDERATIONS FOR INTERNET USE AS A COMMUNICATION TOOL

While a large percentage of Americans are using the Internet for health and non-health reasons, and with the growing popularity of the Internet as a social communications tool, there are several aspects of Internet usage that deserve attention. The first consideration is the use of broadband at home. Broadband connections provide the requisite stability and speeds that enable the social aspects of the Internet and the downloading of basic pages. The most recent data indicate a slowing of broadband adoption, remaining relatively stable at 66%

of American adults (Smith, 2010a). Additionally, 10% of Americans do not have access to broadband. This fact is cause for concern because it suggests that families of lower socioeconomic status may be at a disadvantage when performing basic Internet activities like paying bills, searching for jobs, and searching the Internet in general (Kang, 2011).

The second consideration—termed the "digital divide"—is the disparity between those who have access to information technology and those who do not. In the United States, the proportion of African American or Latino Internet users has almost doubled in the 10 years from 2000 to 2010 (11% to 21%) (Smith, 2010b). Eighty percent of white Americans go online, compared to 71% of African Americans. Looking specifically at home broadband usage, African Americans trail white Americans 56% to 67% (Smith, 2010a). African Americans are also less likely than white Americans to own a desktop computer (51% vs. 65%) (Smith, 2010b). These statistics strongly suggest the presence of a digital divide in the United States.

The third consideration is closely related to the second. While the evidence supports a digital divide characterized by white Americans having greater access than minorities, this is not the case for mobile technology, especially non-voice features of mobile phones. Specifically, minority cell phone owners are more likely than white Americans to use cell phone data applications in 13 activity categories. Additionally, Americans aged 18 to 29 are more likely than those 30 and over to use data applications. However, use of cell phones for data applications is growing among Americans aged 30 to 49. Looking at other forms of mobile access, little variation exists between white Americans, African Americans, and Latinos in laptop ownership and wireless laptop use to access the Internet (Smith, 2010c).

As you continue reading this chapter, you are encouraged to reflect on the considerations above. Keep in mind the similarities and differences in how your patients might access the Internet. Are barriers in place that can impede your ability to communicate with patients? Alternatively, what opportunities exist to enhance communication with patients?

You are also encouraged to visit www.broadbandmap.gov to determine the available broadband providers in your area. Also, visit http://news.bbc.co.uk/2/hi/technology/8552410.stm to see an interesting, interactive depiction of global Internet adoption. Lastly, visit http://www.pewinternet.org/Static-Pages/Trend-Data/Internet-Adoption.aspx to examine specific data regarding Internet adoption in the United States.

Pharmacist Use of Social Media

The term "social media" reflects the second iteration of the Web (i.e., Web 2.0) and is characterized as bidirectional or interactive, dynamic, and utilizing push technologies (Boulos et al., 2006). Another hallmark of social media is user-generated content. Examples of social media you may have heard of, or should consider becoming familiar with, are included in Box 13.3.

Box 13.3 Social Media Categories and Examples

- Videosharing (YouTube, Vimeo, TeacherTube)
- Wikis (Wikipedia, MedPedia, Knol)
- Social networking (Facebook, LinkedIn, hi5)
- Blogs (Blogger, WordPress, Posterous)
- Microblogging (Twitter, tumblr, Yammer)
- Podcasts/vodcasts (iTunes)
- Photosharing (Flickr, Picasa, Photobucket)
- Virtual worlds (Second Life, Visuland)
- Really Simple Syndication (RSS) (Google Reader, Webicina)
- Social bookmarking (delicious, digg, Evernote)
- Location-based services (FourSquare, Facebook Places)
- Platform aggregators (FriendFeed)

Social media is inherently collaborative and can help foster communication. Hence, it is unsurprising that pharmacists are increasingly adopting these tools into their workflow and practice. Social media–mediated delivery of education is also experiencing rapid growth globally in pharmacy (Cain et al., 2010) as well as other specialized applications such as wikis in mental health (Bastida et al., 2010), Anesthesia 2.0 (Chu et al., 2010), and podcasts in cardiology (Santoro, 2008).

Further, these tools can be used both for provider–patient and interprofessional communications. A survey of health care providers in Spain revealed frequent use of the Internet for work-related reasons by pharmacists (93%), physicians (93%), and nurses (74%) (Lupiáñez-Villanueva et al., 2009). Moreover, pharmacists had a blog (16%) more frequently than nurses (9%) or physicians (5%). A study of pharmacists attending a state association meeting found the social media tools most commonly used to be YouTube (74%), Wikipedia (72%), Facebook (50%), and blogs (26%) (Alkhateeb et al., 2011). Separate studies of pharmacy (Cain and Dillon, 2010) and pharmacist (Clauson et al., 2010a) blogs have been conducted, identifying 136 and 44, respectively; the latter also showed that 25% of pharmacist bloggers had a Twitter account.

VIRTUAL PATIENT COMMUNITIES

The same features of social media that enable geographically disparate pharmacists to collaborate offer the same resource to patients. A number of virtual communities have emerged both as self-contained entities and via collections of Web 2.0 tools, like those loosely tying together worldwide communities of patients with diabetes.

Alternately, there are companies trying to help build communities *for* patients, like the Alliance Health Network's resource for diabetics (www.diabeticconnect.com).

Perhaps the most well-known virtual patient community is PatientsLikeMe (www.patientslikeme.com), which was started by three engineers from MIT (Massachusetts Institute of Technology). It also holds the distinction of hosting one of the first reported patient-initiated and -conducted research studies; in this case, the effect of lithium on ALS (Amyotrophic Lateral Sclerosis) (Frost et al., 2008). Two particular aspects of these communities may surprise pharmacists. The first is the meticulous level of detail with which patients record and report disease-related information and treatment. Secondly, because HIPAA was not created to protect patients from self-disclosure, the amount of identifiable patient data that can be accessed on this site can be staggering.

Patient–Provider Communication

Internet-based and other electronic communication between patients and providers offers significant promise through several mechanisms:

1. Health-related content distribution to patients from any Internet-connected device from anywhere in the world
2. Synchronous and asynchronous communication between providers and patients (e.g., telepharmacy, discussion forums, text alerts, etc.)
3. Provision of patient-generated health-related information to their provider
4. Portals that allow patients to access, review, and annotate their medical records
5. Collaborative arrangements using social media tools to help patients manage their medical conditions

The challenge and opportunity of using electronic communication between providers and patients is to identify the technology that best fits the needs of the patient, suits the work flow of the provider, and is most appropriate for the patient's health care need. Ideally, providers and patients will work together to collectively identify the technology, whether one or several tools, that best fit the situation.

Patient–provider electronic communication technology can take many forms. E-mail is one technology that has received considerable attention because of its widespread availability and patients' desire to communicate with their providers (Harris Interactive, 2002; Singh et al., 2009). Despite findings that secure e-mail communication (often through portals) can improve patient outcomes (Zhou et al., 2010), satisfaction (Lin et al., 2005), and communication (Stalberg et al., 2008), barriers remain for its use. Concerns over confidentiality and security often rise to the top in discussions focused on reluctance to use secure e-mail communication (Ye et al., 2010). Additionally, the existence of guidelines for secure patient–provider communication (Kane and Sands, 1998; Zierler-Brown and Pankaskie, 2003) does not necessarily equate to compliance. In fact, one study found a decrease in physicians' interest in e-mailing their patients (Menachemi et al., 2011), and two studies found a decrease in compliance with guidelines (Brooks and Menachemi, 2006; Menachemi et al., 2011).

Despite the starts and stops of e-mail communication between providers and patients, the inclusion of secure patient–physician messaging in the 2010 American Recovery and Reinvestment Act's requirements for meaningful use of electronic health records signals that some form of e-mail communication will likely continue (Zhou et al., 2010).

Beyond e-mail communication, what are you likely to experience as feasible methods to electronically communicate with your patients? The answers are found throughout this chapter and largely center on social media tools, messaging services, and patient-provided information collected during the patient's normal, daily routine.

A recent literature review of the use of health information technology (HIT) for communication between providers and pediatric patients (or their caregivers) requiring follow-up care provides insight into electronic communication. While the review addresses a specific patient population, much of the authors' findings apply to the broad use of HIT to facilitate patient–provider communication (Gentles et al., 2010). In 104 studies, the authors found three broad themes: establishing continuity of care, addressing time constraints, and overcoming geographical barriers. Seven communication methods were used to address the themes: video conference (44% of studies), Internet (33%), telephone (25%), e-mail (21%), manual information download (13%), intranet (6%), and short messaging service (3%). Measured outcomes included clinical outcomes (32% of studies), quality of life (20%), and knowledge (10%). Box 13.4 lists the types of functions performed by the HIT interventions.

Several implications can be found in this review. First, medication management, the primary domain of pharmacists, is the most frequent function, suggesting that opportunities exist for you to become involved in and/or implement electronic communication tools with your patients. Second, the range of communication methods found in the review suggests that you have a variety of options to communicate with your patients. Lastly, physiological monitoring was a frequently performed function. Pharmacists are best able to interpret the importance of physiologic data as it relates to medication therapy. This is an area of opportunity for you to use electronic communication to improve patient outcomes.

Interprofessional Use of Electronic Communication

Electronic methods of communication among health care providers offer the potential for evolutionary changes in the delivery of health care. Providers are using electronic communication tools to (1) enhance or coordinate care of patients and patient populations, (2) disseminate information to peers, (3) influence decision making and behavior, and (4) create or strengthen research collaborations (Cain et al., 2010). These tools include, but are not limited to the following:

- E-mail and listservs
- Text messaging
- Social media
- Telepharmacy

Box 13.4 Health Information Technology Functions in Patient–Provider Electronic Communication

Health-Related Function	Number of Studies (%)
Medication management	49 (47)
Medical consultation	47 (45)
Education	41 (39)
Physiological monitoring	40 (38)
Diagnosis	36 (35)
Caregiver psychological support	34 (33)
Patient behavior management	33 (32)
Professional counseling	33 (32)
Physical care management	18 (17)
Patient psychological support	17 (16)
Behavioral surveillance	16 (15)
Transfer patient data to family	16 (15)
Mental health therapy (noncounseling)	15 (14)
Referral	13 (13)
Virtual family visits	4 (4)

Source: Gentles SJ, Lokker C, McKibbon KA. Health information technology to facilitate communication involving health care providers, caregivers, and pediatric patients: A scoping review. *Journal of Medical Internet Research* 2010. Retrieved February 25, 2011 from http://www.jmir.org/2010/2/e22.

E-MAIL AND LISTSERVS

Research has shown that pharmacists and physicians who are within the same health care system can facilitate communication by using e-mail (Henault et al., 2002). An examination of a wireless, push e-mail system to improve communication in an intensive care unit found reported benefits including improved coordination (88%) and reduced staff frustration (75%) as well as beliefs about faster (90%) and safer (75%) patient care (O'Connor et al., 2009). Unfortunately, use of e-mail among providers related to the care of a patient has the same privacy and system security concerns as use of e-mail between providers and patients. If you send or receive patient information to anyone via your computer, either with computer-generated fax or e-mail, you are required to be HIPAA-compliant.

Use of electronic communication goes beyond communication among providers caring for a patient within a given health care system. For example, radiologists in India may read x-rays, MRIs, or mammograms transmitted from imaging sites in the United States (Lenhart, 2010). Electronic transfer of images using new wireless fidelity systems has evolved such that it now takes <4 seconds, while it previously took nearly 1 hour to transmit a mammogram. Another example is a service for online "second opinions" from specialty experts using physicians from institutions such as Harvard Medical School (Partners Online Specialty Consultations, 2011). E-mail is also used to both disseminate information to fellow health care professionals and influence behavior. The latter was illustrated in a study in which drug information was e-mailed to physicians, resulting in a change in sales of the targeted medication (Edward et al., 2007).

Similarly, e-mail listservs, essentially electronic mailing lists, continue to be thriving tools for connecting pharmacists to fellow providers and excellent sources for posing questions and engaging in discourse (DeWitt et al., 2004). Although LISTSERV is actually the name of specific software, as with Xerox and photocopying, it has grown to be generically associated with the function. In some ways, listservs were an early stage of what is considered social media since it was a method of one-to-many communication.

TEXT MESSAGING

Text messaging is a means of communication using plain text messages that are sent, typically, between mobile devices, although virtually any PC can be used to send and receive them. This mode of communication has gained popularity in recent years, and in 2010, more than 72% of cell phone users reported receiving or sending text messages (Lenhart, 2010). The ascension of "texting" has seen an accompanying decrease in voice conversations, with the average length of a phone call dipping under 2 minutes (U.S. Census Bureau, 2010).

SMS (simple message service) and MMS (multimedia message service) are the two primary classifications of text messages (Henry-Labordère and Jonack, 2004). MMS, as the name implies, also allows communication of data beyond plain text, which can be images, videos, etc. SMS is generally used as an umbrella term and has been used to improve pharmaceutical care via reminders and information about dosage, methods of administration, and adverse drug reactions (Mao et al., 2008) and to collect data (Kew, 2010). SMS also is being used increasingly as a more immediate and informal way to communicate between providers (Olla and Tan, 2009). This trend of immediacy in communication is likely to continue among pharmacists who are members of Generations Y and Z, as 95% of individuals 18 to 29 years old have reported using SMS (Smith, 2010c).

SOCIAL MEDIA

Social media offer a collectively versatile suite of tools for interprofessional communication. Whereas the use of social media (e.g., YouTube, Facebook, Wikipedia, Twitter, Blogger) was discussed earlier in the chapter, specific examples of their application in health care will be explored here and in Case Study 13.1.

CASE STUDY 13.1

Social Networking Sites and Careers

Dr. Reese is a pharmacist who works in a teaching hospital and has connected with others online via the social networking site Facebook for many years. He found that it helped him reconnect with old friends from school and keep up with his widening circle of acquaintances as well. However, newly implemented administrative restructuring and policy changes at his hospital have resulted in a more limited patient care role for him and a restriction from participating in research. As Dr. Reese has increasingly found his job to be less rewarding, he turned to a site aimed at creating professional networking opportunities—LinkedIn. He used LinkedIn to help generate job leads and became more active on PharmQD and Skipta, two social networking sites specifically for pharmacists. He integrated those sites into his job search efforts and was able to obtain an interview at a rural hospital with a pharmacy department interested in transitioning to a more patient-centered approach. Prior to his interview, he searched online and found balanced reviews about the hospital and a blog by a nurse employed there describing a positive partnership with pharmacy.

Upon interviewing at the hospital, one of the hiring managers confided in Dr. Reese that they employed a service that mined data from social media sites for information about potential candidates. Further, the manager revealed they were happy to have found both a lack of negative information about him as well as encouraging signs, such as recommendations about him by former supervisors and peers on LinkedIn. While Dr. Reese felt like the institution was a good fit in many ways, he was worried about the nascent state of research being conducted there along with the institution's geographic isolation. After he expressed those concerns, the hiring manager told him about the NIH (National Institutes of Health)-funded VIVO project (Gewin, 2010), dubbed "Facebook for Scientists." The aim of "Facebook for Scientists" is to create a national network connecting researchers and actively facilitate collaboration.

Lessons Learned

While Dr. Reese still has some difficult decisions to make about his future, he has observed the following:

- Social networking sites can be used effectively for both personal and professional purposes.
- Some hiring managers use information gleaned from searches of social media.
- Actively managing your online digital identity is a responsibility similar to being cognizant of your credit score.
- Social media may be one tool to help improve job satisfaction.
- A job interview starts even before the first formal communication between parties.

Twitter (www.Twitter.com) is a microblogging service in which short bursts of 140-character "tweets" (similar to an SMS) can be transmitted and read by anyone who "follows" them via this social networking hybrid. Some people identify Twitter as simply the status update function of Facebook, but it can be used to accomplish a variety of objectives. Twitter first gained prominence in some people's minds when the U.S. State Department asked that it not be shut down for scheduled maintenance as it was the only open source of communication with Iran during contested elections. It has since been one of the communication and coordination tools used to foment democracy in countries such as Tunisia, Egypt, and Libya (Lee, 2009). Examples of uses in health care include disseminating drug recalls, live tweeting pharmacy conferences, shift bidding among providers, and coordination among first responders (Baumann, 2009).

Among the relatively small number of pharmacists with Twitter accounts identified in 2010, less than half of their tweets (41%) were for health-related purposes (Clauson, 2010b). However, those health-related tweets were frequently used to communicate medical information and to serve as shortened links to original or full sources of information. As an example, Twitter was used to communicate between providers in the following tweet: "Not able to control hypertensive crisis with nitro infusion. Adding nicardepine. I've got only 1 peripheral IV" (Anderson, 2011). In another example, Twitter was used by a community pharmacy to share information with its patients and fellow providers: "H1N1 clinic 10/19/09 1 to 5 P.M. Available only to healthy adults not pregnant 2/24/24 to 49 if contact w/infant > 6 months/ and health care workers" (Rankos Stadium Pharmacy, 2009).

Evernote (www.evernote.com) is a cloud-based application that allows storage of every type of file including PDFs, photos, and web page clips. It can be used as a digital "peripheral brain" like those assembled by many student pharmacists while in school. Evernote also has a social sharing feature that allows the user to share selected files as a notebook either with a selected group or with everyone. One example is a stream of informatics articles curated by a pharmacist at the following site: www.evernote.com/pub/poikonen/PublicPharmacoinformatics.

MedPedia (www.medpedia.com) is similar to the better-known Wikipedia. However, while MedPedia allows anyone to read its medical-themed entries, only credentialed members may contribute articles. It is also a growing social networking space for health care providers and researchers to come together. Later in the chapter, we discuss how social media use may affect the professional persona of a health care provider.

TELEPHARMACY

Telepharmacy is the "provision of all aspects of traditional pharmaceutical care via communication technology to address distances separating participants" (Clauson et al., 2010c). In some states, telemedicine networks are being established to provide consultations in nearly all specialties, including radiology, pathology, oncology, pharmacy, surgery, psychiatry, and behavioral health (Blanchet, 2005). Similarly, telepharmacy has spread to settings ranging from community pharmacies to hospitals (Clauson et al., 2010c). Integrated computer systems give health care professionals access to patient-specific data from a variety of sources and sites of care. Examples of telepharmacy services to remote rural areas or underserved areas of inner cities include automated dispensing at remote sites with no pharmacist present but with a distant, off-site pharmacist "checking" and authorizing the filling of prescriptions. Patients with questions can have audiovisual contact and consultation with the pharmacist at the distant site (Clifton et al., 2003).

As the cost of telepharmacy equipment has fallen and Internet-based videoconferencing options such as Skype (www.skype.com) and ooVoo (www.oovoo.com) have become more available, the use of telepharmacy has accelerated. It has moved from being primarily a remote check-authorize pursuit to offering a fuller scope of pharmacy services. One pharmacy chain has even partnered with American Well to deliver on-demand, fee-based pharmacist services that patients can access from their own home PCs (American Well, 2010).

Trending and Future Electronic Communication Issues

Once considered novel, the use of Internet-based electronic communication tools in health care is becoming the norm. As national adoption and use of the Internet and broadband continue to grow, the opportunities of using electronic communication methods to overcome the challenges of time, distance, and capacity present tangible methods to improve patient care delivery and outcomes. Additionally, national efforts to adopt electronic health records, funded by the federal government, are providing substantial incentives to adopt HIT. While not focused exclusively on the topics covered in this chapter, these federal efforts are important because they are national in scope. It is also very likely that your patients will begin asking for ways to communicate with you electronically, especially as the younger "Millennial" generation moves into the health care system.

Two issues relate to the future of electronic communication, including the provider's experience with these methods. Participatory medicine, self-care, and patient-centered care are becoming common vernacular in today's health care environment. These phrases signify a shift in how health care should be structured. Instead of the provider serving as the dominant expert and the patient as the obedient non-expert, the patient serving as an equal partner with his or her provider will characterize the health care system of the future. The reality is that the patient is the most informed person about his or her health-related experiences and should be actively contributing to his or her medical record and actively involved in determining treatment options. Are providers ready for this shift? Will we see a scenario where patients use an electronic device to capture blood pressure, blood glucose, or some other indicator of health but their providers, including pharmacists, are not willing or able to use this information? If so, the health care system of the future will likely miss an important opportunity to advance care.

The second future issue is the continued importance of confidentiality, privacy, and security of PHI. Some experts have argued that patients' comfort with electronic storage and exchange of their health information is a natural extension of their feelings about online banking, suggesting that patients who are comfortable with online banking will also be comfortable with online health activities. Whereas a bank has insurance that will reimburse an individual if an unscrupulous person accesses their account and illegally acquires their money, no insurance exists to compensate an individual when their personal health details become public knowledge. With many examples of PHI accidentally being made public (iHealthBeat, 2011), the average American is becoming more aware of the risks of using electronic communication technology for health-related activities. To protect PHI, providers should implement actions to protect patient information, discuss with patients the steps they can take to secure their own information, and adopt HIT that is compliant with current standards for secure management of patient information.

Guidelines for Electronic Communications

There are numerous aspects of digital communication that pharmacists should consider. Some considerations are specific to the medium (e.g., e-mail), and others encompass many forms of media (e.g., e-professionalism). This section provides general and specific recommendations for maintaining high levels of clarity and professionalism when communicating online.

E-PROFESSIONALISM

Due to the near ubiquity of conversations that now occur in social media settings, professionals in all fields should familiarize themselves with the concept of e-professionalism. E-professionalism pertains to the online display of traditional professional attitudes and behaviors expected by members of that field (Cain and Romanelli, 2009). A lessening in social restraint (Kiesler et al., 1984) and invisible audiences (Boyd, 2007) are two traits of social media that increase the likelihood that online conversations may result in negative consequences for the author/sender. In traditional face-to-face conversations, individuals are more likely to filter thoughts before expressing them to others. This filtering process is reduced when interacting via computer screens because one does not have to react to facial expressions and verbal replies. Conversations via social media also may be accessible to invisible audiences—people who were not the intended audience but may have access to online posts. These invisible audiences may consist of forgotten social networking connections or viewers made privy to the conversation by others. The nature of social networking is such that many users have more connections than they can cognitively account for and therefore forget about everyone who might be viewing. According to Dunbar (1993), humans are only capable of managing relationships (online or offline) with around 150 people while simultaneously knowing how all those friends relate to each other. In addition, because conversations are digital, they can easily be replicated and sent to anyone with a few quick mouse clicks.

Although many users are careful and cognizant of the attitudes, opinions, and types of information they reveal in online settings, there are numerous instances to the contrary. Unlike others, professionals may be held to higher standards.

While all of us at times may lament about our jobs and the people with whom we come in contact, it behooves those in health care and other professional fields to limit complaints and rants to face-to-face settings outside the public realm.

Research pertaining to pharmacists and social media is relatively new, but reports show that in the context of blogs, several pharmacists have portrayed themselves as complainers and whiners with little empathy for many of the patients in their care (Cain and Dillon, 2010; Clauson et al., 2010a,b). This is not limited to pharmacists, as physicians and other health care providers have also exhibited unprofessional attitudes in the social media environment (Ferdig et al., 2008; Thompson et al., 2008; Chretien et al., 2009).

Regardless of the ethical and/or philosophical arguments surrounding the use of social media posts for judgments of professionalism, many are of the opinion that it is acceptable to review and use information voluntarily published online to judge others' professionalism. This increases the stakes for individuals who may be overlooked for promotions, residency positions, or other honors due to online personas that depict them as unprofessional (Cain et al., 2010).

COMMUNICATING THROUGH SOCIAL MEDIA

Because social media is complex and exhibits characteristics of both public and private conversations, it can be difficult to maintain a professional identity while communicating socially. An individual's personal attitudes, thoughts, and opinions are revealed through channels such as status updates, blog posts, photos, and group affiliations. Traditionally, these aspects of a health care provider's personal life have been considered private and outside the scope of professional consideration. However, because social media information is often open to a much broader and public audience, it may be difficult to separate one's professional attitude from personal attitude. Many may consider this lack of delineation philosophically and/or ethically wrong, but you should use good judgment with the types of information you post online. Both the American Medical Association and the Australian Medical Association, recognizing the complex issues involved with patient communications via social media, have created official policies to guide their members. These policies, found at www.ama-assn.org and www.ama.com.au, provide physicians, residents, and medical students with guidelines for using social media. These guidelines are adaptable to pharmacists in their roles as health care providers.

Basic tips for communicating via social media include the following:

1. Use good judgment when posting information that may anger, humiliate, offend, or mislead others.
2. Consider all *potential* members of the audience and how they might react when you post to a social media site.
3. Avoid frequent posts that may depict you as a whiner or complainer.
4. Avoid any type of post that depicts you as a substance abuser.
5. Understand that many people may be uncomfortable communicating personal information via social media.

6. Do not solicit Facebook friend requests or other social media connections with patients and/or subordinates.
7. When a patient or subordinate makes a Facebook friend request, consider the issues involved with accepting that request.
8. Do not violate patient privacy and confidentiality standards.
9. Do not post sensitive or proprietary information of your employer.
10. Educate yourself on employer expectations regarding employee social media use.
11. When applicable, use privacy features to control access to social media information.
12. Remember that anything posted online may remain there indefinitely.

COMPOSING AND MANAGING E-MAIL MESSAGES

Composing effective e-mail and managing the e-mail process is important to successful communication with patients, coworkers, physicians, and other colleagues. Tips for e-mail communication include the following:

1. Do not use patient names or other identifying information in the e-mail if there is no encryption used.
2. Double-check all "To" fields prior to sending messages.
3. Set up an automatic reply to tell patients or providers that messages were received.
4. Ask patients and providers to acknowledge receipt of messages sent to them.
5. Use an automatic signature with name and full contact information as well as a reminder about the form of communication to use in emergencies.
6. A permanent record of online communications pertinent to treating and monitoring the patient should be maintained as part of the patient record. Perform at least weekly backups of e-mail onto long-term storage.
7. Have written policies on online communications in place to inform staff, colleagues, and patients.
8. Consult with malpractice carriers on plans for e-mail use in patient care.
9. Have a plan in place for evaluating the costs and outcomes of e-mail services (e.g., cost-effectiveness or patient satisfaction).
10. Request that others use a subject line summarizing the content of the message. For example, ask a patient to put "Refill request for Fosamax" into the subject line. This rule also should be followed by the pharmacist in communicating with patients and colleagues as long as encryption and a secure service are used so that PHI is not accessible.
11. Make action requests and time frames for response clear to e-mail recipients.
12. Separate unrelated topics into separate messages, especially if some items deal with more urgent issues than others.
13. Make e-mail messages one page or less if possible.
14. Check e-mail at defined times two to three times a day. Tell people what the schedule is, and let them know that if they need to reach you on short notice, they must use the telephone.

Summary

In order for you to have a meaningful role in patient care in the future, you must be prepared to utilize and even capitalize on the use of emerging technologies and electronic communication capabilities. Most Americans are accustomed to using Internet technologies to make our daily activities more convenient. Online banking, shopping, and communicating with friends and family have become much easier and more efficient with Web-based technologies. It is only natural to expect that individuals would want their health care activities to have the same conveniences, especially when a large portion of those activities occur when they are sick or injured.

It is important that you understand the future demand for Web-based services and become well-versed with the challenges and opportunities that lie ahead. If you wish to begin using e-mail as part of your patient care services, you should carefully examine guidelines established for physicians using e-mail communication in medical practice. Furthermore, when you use social media as part of your professional activities, you should be cognizant of privacy rules, as well as other social media issues such as e-professionalism. The opportunities for utilizing communication technologies to create a better and more efficient health care system exist today. You just need to adapt to the changes they have wrought and take advantage of the opportunities offered.

REVIEW QUESTIONS

1. **What are some new of the new opportunities and challenges of social media and health care?**
2. **What are some ways that pharmacists and patients have used social media?**
3. **What are some of the guidelines for maintaining a professional online persona?**
4. **What "rules" should be used in composing e-mail messages and managing e-mail exchanges?**
5. **Identify two trending issues pertaining to electronic communications.**

REFERENCES

Alkhateeb FM, Clauson KA, Latif DA. Pharmacist use of social media. *International Journal of Pharmacy Practice* 19:5–7, 2011.

American Well. American Well Announces Agreement to Provide Rite Aid With New Pharmacy Service in Select Stores. 2010. Retrieved February 25, 2011 from http://www.americanwell.com/PressRelease_AW_Announces_Agreement_to_Provide_Rite_Aid_With_New_Pharmacy_Service.html.

Anderson PF. Trying to save lives real time via Twitter. Emerging Technologies Librarian, January 13, 2011. Retrieved February 25, 2011 from http://etechlib.wordpress.com/2011/01/13/trying-to-save-lives-in-real-time-via-twitter.

Bastida R, McGrath I, Maude P. Wiki use in mental health practice: Recognizing potential use of collaborative technology. *International Journal of Mental Health Nursing* 19:142–148, 2010.

Baumann P. 140 health care uses for Twitter, January 16, 2009. Retrieved January 11, 2011 from http://philbaumann.com/2009/01/16/140-health-care-uses-for-twitter.

Blanchet J. Innovative programs in telemedicine: The Arizona telemedicine program. *Telemedicine and e-Health* 11:116–123, 2005.

Boulos MN, Maramba I, Wheeler S. Wikis, blogs and podcasts: A new generation of Web-based tools for virtual collaborative clinical practice and education. *BMC Medical Education* 6:41, 2006.

Boyd D. Social network sites: Public, private, or what? 2007. Retrieved July 22, 2009 from http://kt.flexiblelearning.net.au/tkt2007/wp-content/uploads/2007/04/boyd.pdf.

Brooks RG, Menachemi N. Physicians' use of email with patients: Factors influencing electronic communication and adherence to best practices. *Journal of Medical Internet Research*. 2006. Retrieved February 25, 2011 from http://www.jmir.org/2006/1/e2/.

Cain J, Dillon G. Analysis of pharmacy-centric blogs: Types, discourse themes, and issues. *Journal of the American Pharmacists Association* 50:714–719, 2010.

Cain J, Fox BI. Web 2.0 and pharmacy education. *American Journal of Pharmaceutical Education* 73:120, 2009.

Cain J, Romanelli F. E-professionalism: A new paradigm for a digital age. *Currents in Pharmacy Teaching and Learning* 1:66–70, 2009.

Cain J, Romanelli F, Fox B. Pharmacy, social media, and health: Opportunity for impact. *Journal of the American Pharmacists Association* 50:745–751, 2010.

Cain J, Scott DR, Smith K. Use of social media by residency program directors for resident selection. *American Journal of Health-system Pharmacy* 67:1635–1639, 2010.

Chretien KC, Greysen SR, Chretien J-P, et al. Online posting of unprofessional content by medical students. *Journal of American Medical Association* 302:1309–1315, 2009.

Chu LF, Young C, Zamora A, et al. Anesthesia 2.0: Internet-based information resources and Web 2.0 applications in anesthesia education. *Current Opinion in Anaesthesiology* 23:218–227, 2010.

Clauson KA, Elkins J, Goncz CE. Use of blogs by pharmacists. *American Journal of Health-system Pharmacy* 67:2043–2048, 2010a.

Clauson KA, Ramos Y, Morejon Y, Hawker MD. Analysis of a national sample of pharmacist generated Twitter content [3-073]. American Society of Health-System Pharmacists Midyear Clinical Meeting, Anaheim, CA, December 2010b.

Clauson KA, Seamon MJ, Fox BI. Pharmacists' duty to warn in the age of social media. *American Journal of Health-System Pharmacy* 67:1290–1293, 2010c.

Clifton GD, Byer H, Heaton K, et al. Provision of pharmacy services to underserved populations via remote dispensing and two-way videoconferencing. *American Journal of Health-System Pharmacy* 60:2577–2582, 2003.

DeWitt AL, Gunn SR, Hopkins P, et al. Critical care medicine mailing list: Growth of an online forum. *British Medical Journal* 328:1180, 2004.

Dunbar RI. Coevolution of neocortical size, group size and language in humans. *Behavioral and Brain Sciences* 16:681–735, 1993.

Edward C, Himmelmann A, Wallerstedt SM. Influence of an e-mail with a drug information attachment on sales of prescribed drugs: A randomized controlled study. *BMC Clinical Pharmacology* 7, 2007.

Eysenbach G. Medicine 2.0: Social networking, collaboration, participation, apomediation, and openness. *Journal of Medical Internet Research*. 2008. Retrieved February 25, 2011 from http://www.jmir.org/2008/3/e22/.

Fashner J, Drye ST. Internet availability and interest in patients at a family medical residency clinic. *Family Medicine* 43:117–120, 2011.

Ferdig R, Dawson K, Black EW, et al. Medical students' and residents' use of online social networking tools: Implications for teaching professionalism in medical education. First Monday. 2008. Retrieved September 24, 2010 from http://firstmonday.org/htbin/cgiwrap/bin/ojs/index.php/fm/article/viewArticle/2161/2026.

Fox B. The Internet. In Felkey BG, Fox BI, Thrower MR (eds.). *Health Care Informatics: A Skills-Based Resource* (pp. 109–129). Washington, DC: American Pharmacists Association, 2005.

Fox S. Health topics. February 2, 2011. Retrieved February 25, 2011 from http://pewinternet.org/reports/2011/healthtopics.aspx.

Freudenheim M. Digital Rx: Take two aspirins and email me in the morning. March 2, 2005. Retrieved February 24, 2011 from http://www.nytimes.com/2005/03/02/technology/02online.html.

Frost JH, Massagli MP, Wicks P, et al. How the social web supports patient experimentation with a new therapy: The demand for patient-controlled and patient-centered informatics. *AMIA Annual Symposium Proceedings* 217–221, 2008.

Gentles SJ, Lokker C, McKibbon KA. Health information technology to facilitate communication involving health care providers, caregivers, and pediatric patients: A scoping review. *Journal of Medical Internet Research* 2010. Retrieved February 25, 2011 from http://www.jmir.org/2010/2/e22/.

Gewin V. Collaboration: Social networking seeks critical mass. *Nature* 468:993–994, 2010.

Harris Interactive. Patient/Physician online communication: Many patients want it, would pay for it, and it would influence their choice of doctors and health plans. Health Care News [serial on the Internet]. April 10, 2002. Retrieved February 27, 2011 from http://harrisinteractive.com/news/newsletters/healthnews/HI_health carenews2002vol2_iss08.pdf.

Henault RG, Eugenio KR, Kelliher AF, et al. Transmitting clinical recommendations for diabetes care via e-mail. *American Journal of Health-System Pharmacy* 59:2166–2169, 2002.

Henry-Labordère A, Jonack V. SMS and MMS Interworking in Mobile Networks. Boston, MA: Artech House, Inc., 2004.

Heussner KM. Timeline: Internet turns 40 today…or does it? September 2, 2009. Retrieved February 27, 2011 from http://abcnews.go.com/Technology/story?id=8466876.

iHealthBeat.com. Breaches hit nearly five million in year one after HITECH Act. February 25, 2011. Retrieved February 27, 2011 from http://www.ihealthbeat.org/articles/2011/2/25/breaches-hit-nearly-five-million-in-year-one-after-hitech-act.aspx.

Kane B, Sands DZ. Guidelines for the clinical use of electronic mail with patients. *Journal of the American Medical Informatics Association*. 5:104–111, 1998.

Kang C. Internet service map data show no broadband access for up to 10% in U.S. February 17, 2011. Retrieved February 26, 2011 from http://voices.washingtonpost.com/posttech/2011/02/the_federal_government_on_thur.html.

Kiesler S, Siegel J, McGuire TW. Social psychological aspects of computer-mediated communication. *American Psychologist* 39:1123–1134, 1984.

Kew S. Text messaging: An innovative method of data collection in medical research. *BMC Research Notes* 3:342, 2010.

Lee M. Officials: Twitter Stayed Online for Iran Chaos. Associated Press, Washington, June 16, 2009.

Lee TB. How it all started. 2004. Retrieved February 25, 2011 from http://www.w3.org/2004/Talks/w3c10-HowItAllStarted/.

Leiner BM, Cerf VG, Clark DD, et al. A brief history of the Internet. 2010. Available at: http://www.isoc.org/internet/history/brief.shtml. Accessed February 27, 2011.

Lenhart, A. Cell Phones and American Adults. Pew Internet & American Life Project, September 2, 2010. Retrieved February 25, 2011 from http://www.pewinternet.org/~/media//Files/Reports/2010/PIP_Adults_Cellphones_Report_2010.pdf.

Liederman EM, Morefield CS. Web messaging: A new tool for patient-physician communication. *Journal of the American Medical Informatics Association* 10:260–270, 2003.

Lightspeed Research. Consumers would embrace email communication with their doctor. September 29, 2009. Retrieved February 25, 2011 from http://www.lightspeedresearch.com/pdf/LSR_PR_ConsumersWouldEmbraceEmailCommunication.pdf.

Lin CT, Wittevrongel L, Moore L, et al. An Internet-based patient-provider communication system: Randomized controlled trial. *Journal of Medical Internet Research*. 2005. Retrieved February 25, 2011 from http://www.jmir.org/2005/4/e47/.

Lupiáñez-Villanueva F, Mayer MA, Torrent J. Opportunities and challenges of Web 2.0 within the health care systems: An empirical exploration. *Informatics for Health and Social Care* 34: 117–126, 2009.

Mao Y, Zhang Y, Zhai S. Mobile phone text messaging for pharmaceutical care in a hospital in China. *Journal of Telemedicine and Telecare* 14(8):410–414, 2008.

Menachemi N, Prickett C, Brooks R. The use of physician-patient email: A follow-up examination of adoption and best practice adherence 2005–2008. *Journal of Medical Internet Research*. 2011. Retrieved February 24, 2011 from http://www.jmir.org/2011/1/e23/.

Merriam-Webster. Definition: killer app. Retrieved February 26, 2011 from http://www.merriam-webster.com/dictionary/killer%20app.

O'Connor C, Friedrich JO, Scales DC, et al. The use of wireless e-mail to improve health care team communication. *Journal of the American Medical Informatics Association* 16:705–713, 2009.

Olla P, Tan J (eds.). *Mobile Health Solutions for Biomedical Applications*. Hershey, PA: Medical Information Science Reference, 2009.

Partners Online Speciality Consultations. Harvard Medical School, 2011. Retrieved June 7, 2011 from https://econsults.partners.org/v2/(mr0pqn45timdd25524nujw45)/default.aspx.

Pew Internet. Trend data. September 2010. Retrieved February 26, 2011 from http://www.pewinternet.org/Trend-Data/Online-Activities-Daily.aspx.

Rankos Stadium Pharmacy. Twitter Account, October 18, 2009. Available at: http://twitter.com/rankos-pharmacy. Accessed October 18, 2009.

Santoro E. Using podcasts for the cardiologist's education and update. [abstract]. *Recenti Progressi in Medicina* 99:163–170, 2008.

Singh H, Fox SA, Petersen N, et al. Older patients' enthusiasm to use electronic mail to communicate with their physicians: Cross-sectional survey. *Journal of Medical Internet Research*. 2009. Retrieved February 24, 2011 from http://www.jmir.org/2009/2/e18/.

Sittig DF, King S, Hazelhurst BL. A survey of patient-provider e-mail communication: What do patients think? *International Journal of Medical Informatics* 61(1):71–80, 2001.

Smith A. Home broadband 2010. August 22, 2010a. Retrieved February 24, 2011 from http://www.pewinternet.org/Reports/2010/Home-Broadband-2010.aspx.

Smith A. Technology trends among people of color. September 17, 2010b. Retrieved February 25, 2011 from http://www.pewinternet.org/Commentary/2010/September/Technology-Trends-Among-People-of-Color.aspx.

Smith A. Mobile access 2010. Pew Internet & American Life Project, July 7, 2010c. Retrieved February 26, 2011 from http://www.pewinternet.org/~/media//Files/Reports/2010/PIP_Mobile_Access_2010.pdf.

Stalberg P, Yeh M, Ketteridge G, et al. E-mail access and improved communication between patient and surgeon. *Archives of Surgery* 2008. Retrieved February 25, 2011 from http://archsurg.ama-assn.org/cgi/reprint/143/2/164.

Thompson LA, Dawson K, Ferdig R, et al. The intersection of online social networking with medical professionalism. *Journal of General Internal Medicine* 23:954–957, 2008.

U.S. Census Bureau. Statistical Abstract of the United States. 2010. Section 24 Information and Communications. Retrieved February 25, 2011 from http://www.census.gov/prod/2009pubs/10statab/infocomm.pdf.

Ward M. How the web went world wild. August 3, 2006. Retrieved February 25, 2011 from http://news.bbc.co.uk/2/hi/technology/5242252.stm.

Ye J, Rust G, Fry-Johnson Y, et al. E-mail in patient-provider communication: A systematic review. *Patient Education and Counseling* 80:266–273, 2010.

Zierler-Brown S, Pankaskie M. Guidelines for provider-patient email. *Journal of the American Pharmacists Association* 42:737–738, 2003.

Zhou YY, Kanter MH, Wang JJ, et al. Improved quality at Kasier Permanente through e-mail between physicians and patients. *Health Affairs* 29:1370–1375, 2010.

CHAPTER

14

Ethical Behavior When Communicating with Patients

MONA M. SEDRAK

Overview

This chapter outlines how the changing world of health care has created ethical dilemmas for pharmacists and how an ethical framework is often needed to guide behavior when communicating with patients. The Ethical Code of Conduct for Pharmacists drafted by the American Pharmaceutical Association (APhA) is discussed, and key ethical principles that apply to the delivery of pharmaceutical care and medication therapy management (MTM) are introduced. A structured guide for moral decision making and ethical case resolution also is presented. Case studies and corresponding analyses are included to help readers apply skills in ethical case resolution. Finally, several contemporary topics that are causing national concern and making headlines for today's pharmacists are discussed.

Ethical Patient Care

The following Case Studies 14.1 to 14.3 illustrate several principles of ethical behavior. As you read, make notes about what you would do in each situation. At the end of the chapter, you will find an analysis of each case. Before reading the

CASE STUDY 14.1

Ms. Edwards is starting on a new medication for schizophrenia. The drug has a number of side effects, some of which can be serious. She asks you several questions about the purpose of the medication and possible side effects. When you ask her what her physician told her about the medication, she reports that he said, "I've got a lot of patients on this drug and they're doing fine." It is obvious to you that she is unclear about the purpose of the medication or any possible problems. You are concerned that Ms. Edwards may refuse to take the drug if told about possible side effects. What would you say to Ms. Edwards?

CASE STUDY 14.2

James Bently, a 17-year-old patient of your pharmacy, was diagnosed with epilepsy and prescribed phenytoin about 6 months ago. In conversations with him, you have discovered that he considers epilepsy embarrassing and has indicated he does not believe his physician is correct in the diagnosis. James expressed his belief that he does not really need the drug. Your refill records indicate a pattern of nonadherence to the medication. In the past, you have tried to educate him about phenytoin and the importance of consistent use in controlling seizures. However, he still does not take the drug as prescribed. James also continues to drive his car, and you are aware that he was recently charged in a noninjury automobile accident. His father, who occasionally picks up the medication for James, has never indicated awareness of his son's denial of epilepsy or nonadherence with treatment. Should you disclose the fact that James is not taking his medication to his father? To his physician? To the police?

CASE STUDY 14.3

You are working as a relief pharmacist in a community pharmacy. You notice that Megan, the 17-year-old daughter of a very close family friend, is receiving prescriptions for oral contraceptives and for the treatment of a sexually communicated infection (SCI). Apparently, Megan has been hanging out with a group of students whom her parents disapprove of and have forbidden her to see. You are very concerned about Megan and wonder whether her use of oral contraceptives may lead her to forgo the use of condoms that could offer protection from SCIs. When Megan enters the pharmacy to pick up her prescriptions, she becomes upset at seeing you and hurries out, refusing to talk to you. You know that if you were in her parents' shoes, you would want to know about the prescriptions. You are convinced that Megan is in trouble and needs the help of her family.

analyses, reread the cases and see if you would resolve them any differently than you initially thought. Then compare your analyses with those provided.

Each of these cases presents decisions that must be made on the basis of legal and ethical principles. The legal aspects of these cases are covered under state and federal law. However, many elements of how a professional should behave are not addressed in laws and regulations, but are covered by underlying ethical principles of patient–health professional relationships. Thus, your ability to choose a proper course of action in these situations depends on your understanding of the ethical principles involved, especially in the areas of beneficence, nonmalfeasance (i.e., doing no harm), autonomy, and honesty. Other issues that follow from these principles and are particularly important in patient counseling are informed consent, confidentiality, and fidelity. These important concepts will be discussed in later sections of this chapter.

A Pharmacy Code of Conduct for a Modern World

Over the last few decades, rapid advancements in health care and adoption of new technologies have changed the environment in which health care is rendered. Despite these changes, health care remains an exciting and complex arena offering rich opportunities for growth, professional satisfaction, and interesting intellectual challenges that affect all of its professionals—including pharmacists. The emerging role of pharmacists in MTM requires pharmacists to be more effective and efficient when engaging in all forms of communication related to medication (Dhillon et al., 2001). The ability-based outcomes expected of graduating pharmacists as set forth by the Accreditation Council for Pharmaceutical Education Standards (2007) states that "standards focus on the development of students'… sound and reasoned judgment and the highest level of ethical behavior." Thus, it is not uncommon to see pharmacy schools and colleges articulating their desire to graduate pharmacists who are capable of demonstrating "the professional attitudes, habits, and values required to provide ethical and compassionate patient care for the benefit of the individual and community being served" (VCU, 2010).

As the delivery of comprehensive pharmaceutical care grows, you and your staff will find yourselves dealing with a vast array of ethical and legal considerations and challenges. You will need to resolve these if you are to deliver on the promise of providing more cognitive services or simply "helping people get the best use of their medicine." This nine-word phrase was adopted by the Joint Commission of Pharmacy Practitioners following its Pharmacy in the 21st Century Conference (Zellmer, 2001; Tindall and Millonig, 2003) as a simple attempt to convey the complex reasoning behind the MTM movement. This "helping people" approach, which involves beneficent acts, means you will do more than dispense prescriptions. Because your practice sites also will serve as repositories of sensitive and protected health information (PHI), you may become involved in contemporary social issues such as provision of medications that end life or situations that involve terminating pregnancies (see Case Study 14.4) or never starting pregnancies ("morning after" medicines or birth control). Thus, you must be prepared

CASE STUDY 14.4

Nancy, a 16-year-old student, presents a prescription for Plan B, which is used for emergency postcoital contraception. The pharmacist on duty, Jeff, is a strong pro-life supporter and refuses to fill the prescription. Nancy becomes very upset and pleads with Jeff to fill the prescription as this is the only pharmacy near campus that accepts her insurance and she does not have any means of getting to another pharmacy. Nancy tearfully explains to Jeff that the reason she needs the prescription is that she was attacked and raped walking back to her dorm from a party. Jeff stands firm and recommends that Nancy seek counseling. The patient leaves the pharmacy without the prescription in a very agitated and emotional state. The day after she calls and speaks to Jeff's manager, explains the situation, and demands that Jeff be fired. Did Jeff have the right to refuse to dispense the medication? What was Jeff's duty to the patient?

to recognize and resolve ethical issues by understanding ethical principles and applying them to the delivery of pharmaceutical care and MTM.

The Pharmacists' Code of Ethics

The APhA adopted a revised Code of Ethics for Pharmacists in 1994; the American Society of Health-System Pharmacists (ASHP) endorsed this code in 1996. Using a patient-centered approach, the code's eight principles are based on moral obligations and virtues intended to guide pharmacists in their professional relationships with patients and other health care professionals (APhA, 1994). This pharmacist-specific Code of Ethics addresses only ethical behavior and does not address any state and federal statutes and regulations governing pharmacy practice. However, such statutes and regulations also address how pharmacists are to conduct themselves in relationships designed to respect and protect the well-being of the public. The eight principles described in the APhA Code of Ethics for Pharmacists are as follows:

I. A pharmacist respects the covenantal relationship between the patient and pharmacist.
II. A pharmacist promotes the good of every patient in a caring, compassionate, and confidential manner.
III. A pharmacist respects the autonomy and dignity of each patient.
IV. A pharmacist acts with honesty and integrity in professional relationships.
V. A pharmacist maintains professional competence.
VI. A pharmacist respects the values and abilities of colleagues and other health professionals.
VII. A pharmacist serves individual, community, and societal needs.
VIII. A pharmacist seeks justice in the distribution of health resources.

While these principles outline pharmacists' professional obligation to use their knowledge and skills for the benefit of others, they reflect general and ethical principles held in high esteem by all health care professionals. Many pharmacy schools have articulated them in their codes of conduct. For example, the regents of a well-known university have approved a document stating that graduates of its School of Pharmacy will exhibit "the highest standards of professional and ethical behavior in pharmacy practice" and names seven behaviors its graduates must possess: (a) honesty, (b) integrity, (c) tolerance, (d) confidentiality, (e) care and compassion, (f) respect for others, and (g) responsibility. However, and just as importantly, the APhA Code of Ethics was built on how contemporary society interprets underlying ethical principles that have guided mankind for millennia. The principles articulated in the Code of Ethics are: (a) nonmalfeasance, (b) beneficence, (c) autonomy, (d) honesty and truth-telling, (e) informed consent, (f) confidentiality, and (g) fidelity. These principles (see Box 14.1) are something every pharmacist should understand and incorporate into his or her committed lifestyle as a professional.

Key Principles Guiding Ethical Conduct

THE PRINCIPLE OF NONMALFEASANCE

The "principle of nonmalfeasance" is derived from the Latin maxim "*primum non nocere*" (first, do no harm), which has been taught to medical students as the moral maxim that had its beginnings 3,500 years ago in the Oath of Hippocrates. The principle of nonmalfeasance requires a health care provider to not act in any way that intentionally inflicts needless harm or injury to a patient, either through acts of commission or omission (Munson, 2000). Most health professionals take a utilitarian approach by deciding whether an action will do the greatest good over using another course of action. Pharmacists must always be aware of the drugs they are dispensing and the advice they give people when there is potential for that treatment to cause harm.

The principle of nonmalfeasance can be violated in two distinct ways. First, pharmacists can violate this principle if they knowingly and intentionally cause

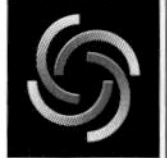

Box 14.1 Underlying Ethical Principles

- Nonmalfeasance
- Beneficence
- Autonomy
- Honesty and truth-telling
- Informed consent
- Confidentiality
- Fidelity

a patient harm. For example, knowingly filling a prescription to which a patient has an allergy or filling a prescription in defiance of the published literature that states it will have a drug–food interaction without telling the patient about the drug–food interaction may be interpreted as malfeasance. The principle of nonmalfeasance may also be violated when no malice or intent to do harm is involved. This would include situations where unintentional harms result from negligence.

For example, a pharmacist mistakenly reads a prescription for Zyrtec and fills it with Zyprexa. Should that patient come to harm through this error, the pharmacist may be found negligent in his or her actions even though the pharmacist had no intention to cause harm. The pharmacist may be considered as having failed "to exercise a standard of due care" in discharging his or her responsibilities as a professional. Thus, the pharmacist failed to meet his or her obligation of nonmalfeasance and may be held accountable by a court system for his or her actions. The obligation of care imposed by the principle of nonmalfeasance is not to demand that pharmacists or any health professional accomplish the impossible or be perfect in any way. Rather, pharmacists must provide a standard of care that any reasonable professional would have provided under the same or similar circumstances and at a level higher than an "ordinary" person. In essence, this expectation is reasonable because perfection in medicine is not possible since it is not a perfect or exact science. Thus, pharmacists and other health care professionals are held to "standards of due care." It is by these standards, set by the professional behavior of equals, that actions are evaluated and judged as either harmful or appropriate.

To further protect members of society from "malfeasance," the following types of standards have been established:

a. Licensing statutes and regulations
b. Educational requirements for entry into the profession
c. Continuing professional education standards for assurance of practical learning skills
d. Credentialing bodies or committees that set up entry barriers to a professional curriculum or specialty

Through these means, society has some assurance that individuals trained as pharmacists have obtained, and hopefully continue to maintain, an acceptable level of knowledge and skills necessary for them to take on the public trust of providing pharmaceutical care. Thus, the APhA Code of Ethics for Pharmacists addresses the ethical principle of nonmalfeasance when it states that pharmacists must maintain professional competence and that they "have a duty to maintain knowledge and abilities as new medication, devices, and technologies become available and health information advances."

THE PRINCIPLE OF BENEFICENCE

"As to disease, make a habit of two things—to help or at least to do no harm." This directive from the writings of Hippocrates focuses on two moral principles: nonmalfeasance, as discussed above, and beneficence. Both principles require the health care provider to evaluate the potential benefits of an intervention in relation to its risk of harming a patient. Beneficence is the ethical principle that health professionals should behave in the best interest of those they serve. The principle of beneficence is also addressed in the APhA Code of Ethics for Pharmacists (APhA, 1994) when it states, "a pharmacist places concern for the well-being of the patient at the center of professional practice." Thus, when considering a medical or pharmaceutical intervention, including patient educational activities, that intervention should answer some or all of the following questions:

1. Does it promote health and prevent disease?
2. Does it relieve symptoms, pain, and suffering?
3. Does it cure the disease?
4. Will it prevent untimely death?
5. Will it improve functional status or maintain a current health state?
6. Will it help better a patient's condition and prognosis?
7. Will it help avoid harm to the patient in the course of care (e.g., promote patient safety)?

Although there are times when all or most of these questions can be answered, there are times in every professional's life when it is difficult to accomplish a desired therapeutic outcome due to a conflict between patient and provider expectations (i.e., what patients "want" versus what a professional thinks they "need") (Jonsen et al., 2002). For example, the use of combined antiretroviral therapy in the treatment of HIV infection comes with many benefits as well as risks. While the use of these drugs improves patients' quality of life and prolongs their survival, the side-effect profiles of these drugs are extensive, and the cost for the drugs may be extremely burdensome to patients. Thus, the use of these drugs produces a risk-to-benefit relationship that must be carefully considered by both patient and practitioner.

THE PRINCIPLE OF AUTONOMY

Another ethical issue in health care is based on the possible conflict between patient autonomy (the right to make decisions on personal health care) and providers' sense of paternalism in relationships with patients. Paternalistic providers see themselves in a parental role believing they know what is best for their "child" (i.e., patient). In essence, paternalism is a poor practice as it fails to take into consideration the preferences, beliefs, and practices of patients, especially those that could be of most benefit to them. Yet, there are times when patients' preferences are unknown because of their incapacity to express them. Conversely, the principle of autonomy establishes patients' rights to self-determination, that is, the right of patients to choose their own life plans and courses of action (Munson, 2000; Jonsen et al., 2002). This right is considered paramount even if health professionals judge patient decisions as being damaging to their health. According to the "Do No Harm Principle" (i.e., nonmalfeasance), constraints on an individual's free choices are morally permissible only when an individual's preference infringes on the rights and welfare of others (Munson, 2000).

When pharmacists want to assess situations involving ethical dilemmas, they find it helpful to do this in light of a patient autonomy–paternalistic provider continuum. If they assess some provider actions as being more authoritarian than others, they would place these actions toward the "paternalistic" end of this continuum. Actions that encourage patient involvement in decision making would be placed toward the "patient autonomy" end of this continuum. In daily practice, however, there may be many forces that limit or even obstruct the appreciation of patient autonomy, such as the possibly compromised competence of patients, the disparity between provider and patient knowledge, and the stresses that illness can place on patient ability to make decisions (Jonsen et al., 2002).

Medical ethicists often state that the danger of paternalism is that it threatens individual rights and personal liberties. Yet, in past times, medicine has used the beneficence principle as justification for "paternalistic" relationships with patients. For example, physicians made decisions by themselves (without necessarily informing patients and without patient consent) and then did what was necessary because they saw it as in the patient's best interest. Put another way, they made certain decisions based on their perceptions of what was needed, and they did not include the patient in their decision making. Similarly, pharmacists say they are using "professional judgment" when they contact a physician to suggest that a patient's medications be changed without asking the patient first, rationalizing that the patient has no need to know what has happened.

Although most health care professionals embrace and find value in the principle of patient autonomy, in some situations patient autonomy may be unintentionally compromised. For example, patients who are shy, nonassertive, uneducated, or illiterate may be intimidated in the presence of anyone wearing a white coat. Thus, although the pharmacist is not deliberately attempting to infringe on the patient's autonomy, social and psychosocial factors may be so overpowering that the patient feels he or she is powerless to make a decision.

It is easy to see how autonomy is critically linked to information. Information is vital to protecting and preserving patient autonomy. In an era of consumer-driven health care, it is hard to deny patients an active partnership role in their health care. This active decision-making role requires well-informed patients. Likewise, to become well-informed, patients need to be given information in language they understand and to have providers explain in unbiased terms the possible treatment options, risks, and benefits. In today's hurried medical environment, patient education and even informed consent often are pushed aside. Patients often feel rushed and unprepared to make important decisions about their health care and thus relinquish their right to autonomy to their provider.

One case illustrating these principles is the debate over physicians and pharmacists who refuse to prescribe or dispense emergency contraceptives. On one hand, you have those who believe that health professionals should not have to engage in practices to which they have moral objections, while others believe that patients should have access to any and all legal treatments even if their physicians and pharmacists are troubled by their requests. Such issues are bound to raise questions about the balance of rights between patients and their health care providers (Curlin et al., 2007).

THE PRINCIPLE OF HONESTY AND TRUTH-TELLING

Communications between patients and their health professionals should be truthful. But what should be done when full disclosure of every detail could prove to be harmful? With the increased prominence of the principle of autonomy and patients' right to the information necessary to provide informed consent, full disclosure and truthfulness have become the more accepted ethical courses of action (Jonsen et al., 2002; Da Silva et al., 2003).

The principle of honesty requires that patients have the right to truthful communication regarding their medical condition, course of their disease, treatments recommended, and alternative treatments available. The APhA Code of Ethics (1994) states that a pharmacist "has a duty to tell the truth and to act with conviction of conscience." A certain level of trust must develop between patients and pharmacists. This trust is developed when pharmacists adhere to the principle of honesty. Pharmacists appear to be doing a good job in this arena as nearly three-quarters of Americans rate them as having very high or high honesty and ethical standards (Gallup Poll, 2009).

Some health care providers, when withholding information, will claim "therapeutic privilege" as their reason for doing so. This is because they perceive that full disclosure of all medical information would be harmful or upsetting to the patient. In addition, "therapeutic privilege" supports those who base ethical behavior on a paternalistic viewpoint of knowing what is best for the patient. However, this "runs contrary to respect for patient autonomy" (Veatch, 2000). Further, therapeutic privilege, as a paternalistic attitude, has been criticized because "displaying such behavior is not seen as providing a service but as guarding special knowledge and who would be in control as to when and who to reveal the truth to" (Da Silva et al., 2003).

Pharmacists may find themselves in the middle of an ethical dilemma concerning truth-telling and therapeutic privilege. For example, a patient who claims to have allergies and/or hypersensitivities to medications previously taken may be prescribed a similar medication because a prescribing provider believes the problem is not really an allergic reaction. In some cases, the patient's pharmacist may be asked to withhold a patient drug information sheet. The prescribing provider may claim "therapeutic privilege," stating that telling the patient of possible side effects or adverse reactions may cause the patient undue distress or lead to the patient not taking the medication at all. This leaves the pharmacist in a position to make his or her decision not only within the confines of statutes and regulations, but also under his or her own interpretation of what is ethically acceptable.

THE PRINCIPLE OF INFORMED CONSENT

"Informed consent is a critical element of any theory that gives weight to autonomy" (Veatch, 2000). Thus, "informed consent" is the way in which patient preferences become expressed and are applied out of respect for that patient's autonomy (Jonsen et al., 2002). Both honesty and autonomy serve as foundations to the right of the patient to give informed consent to treatment. The informed consent principle states that patients have the right to full disclosure of all relevant aspects of care and must give deliberate consent to treatment based on "usable" information and a clear understanding of that information (Munson, 2000; Quallich, 2005). In general, consent is not required when a procedure is simple and the risks are commonly understood (Cady, 2000). However, any provider who recommends treatment for a patient, especially if it is invasive, must engage in a process that assures that the patient has provided informed consent. The process involves a dialogue between provider and patient focused on the risks and benefits of treatment options, including details such as recovery time. The patient then signs a document intended to provide evidence that he or she understood what was explained during the process of obtaining informed consent.

Informed consent forms the ethical basis for the patient–provider relationship as it "consists of an encounter characterized by mutual participation, good communication, mutual respect, and shared decision making" (Jonsen et al., 2002). For informed consent to successfully take place, it requires a dialogue between patient and provider that consists of the following five distinct components (Quallich, 2005):

- Diagnosis or nature of the specific condition that requires treatment(s)
- The purpose and distinct nature of the treatment(s)
- Risks and potential complications associated with the proposed treatment(s)
- All reasonable alternative treatment(s) or procedures and a discussion of their relative risks and benefits, including the option of taking no action
- The probability of success of the proposed treatment(s)

Thus, it is understood that informed consent has occurred and treatment can be implemented if all relevant information is provided, if consent is freely given without coercion, and if the patient understands the salient information provided.

Even under the best of circumstances, it is not always easy to determine who is competent to consent to treatment and who is not (Munson, 2000; Wingfield, 2003). Health care providers must consider how "vulnerable populations," such as children, those who are cognitively impaired, and those suffering from psychiatric illnesses, are to be considered with respect to consent. The law often uses the terms "competence" and "incompetence" to indicate whether individuals have the legal authority to make health care decisions for themselves. Judges alone have the authority to rule that an individual is legally incompetent. However, medical providers may encounter legally competent patients who appear to have their mental capacity compromised by illness, anxiety, pain, or even hospitalization (Jonsen et al., 2002; Wingfield, 2003). This clinical situation is referred to as "decisional capacity" rather than the legal term of "determination of competency."

Many times in actual practice, health care professionals focus more on "disclosure" than on patient understanding of information (Beauchamp, 1989). Communication between patients and pharmacists must focus on patients' understanding of crucial information that may affect their health care decisions. The pharmacist must create an atmosphere that encourages patients to seek answers to questions. Unfortunately, this style of dialogue is often inhibited by pharmacists' inability to listen carefully to their patient's words and underlying emotions and by time constraints imposed by reimbursement policies that reward procedures rather than education (Jonsen et al., 2002).

A meaningful dialogue or consent process is unlikely to be initiated by patients for a variety of reasons. This is true in part because of patient reticence to question providers. In addition, patients often do not know when there is important information about treatment that they have not yet acquired. The burden is on providers to make sure patients understand all they need to know both to make a reasoned decision about therapy and to implement therapeutic plans appropriately.

While drug therapy is the most common type of therapy in health care, informed consent issues surrounding drug therapy are largely ignored compared with issues involving other types of treatment, such as surgery. In addition, patients have much more control over their decision to adhere or not adhere to their medication therapy. Earlier assumptions by society that risks associated with drug therapy are minimal have been challenged by research reports, such as the Institute of Medicine's *Crossing the Quality Chasm* (IOM, 2001). The estimated number of deaths and adverse health events caused by inappropriate drug therapy is staggering. In the future, pharmacists will be expected to assume their share of responsibility in ensuring that informed consent has occurred before drug treatment is initiated.

What role may pharmacists play in the informed consent process? Many pharmacists assume that when patients bring in prescriptions, (a) their physicians have provided all relevant information, (b) patients understand the information, and (c) they have consented to treatment. In fact, many patients lack information on crucial aspects of drug treatment. In addition, physicians frequently do not explicitly discuss key aspects of drug therapy and often fail to obtain meaningful consent from patients.

In certain situations, it may become clear that informed consent has not occurred. Patients may not fully understand important aspects of treatment, may have unanswered questions, or may not be aware of significant side effects. In addition, patients may indicate reluctance to begin taking medications but feel they have no choice but to follow their physicians' directions. Many may feel coerced into their decision based on the hierarchical relationship between patient and provider, where power is largely vested in the health professionals on whom patients feel dependent. It is difficult to determine whether consent to treatment has been freely given. When patients express reservations about initiating drug treatment, pharmacists may need to consult not only with patients but also with prescribing physicians to discuss the lack of genuine informed consent to treatment.

THE PRINCIPLE OF CONFIDENTIALITY

The Hippocratic Oath states, "what I may see or hear in or outside the course of treatment… which on no account must be spread abroad, I will keep to myself, holding such things shameful to speak about." The principle of confidentiality serves to ensure that health care providers are obligated to refrain from divulging information obtained from patients during medical treatment and to take reasonable precautions to protect that information. Regarding confidentiality, "modern medical ethics bases this duty on respect for the autonomy of the patient, on the loyalty owed by the physician, and on the possibility that disregard of confidentiality would discourage patients from revealing useful diagnostic information and encourage others to use medical information to exploit patients" (Jonsen et al., 2002).

As pharmacists become more involved with direct patient care, they gain access to a wide range of sensitive and private patient information, which is necessary for appropriately managing therapy. With the advent of regulations set by the Health Insurance Portability and Accountability Act of 1996 (HIPAA), pharmacists must know the workings of this statute and be able to address issues relating to confidentiality and consent, as well as regulations concerning "PHI." This new layer of professional responsibility is made all the more important because the greatest challenges to confidentiality today result from technological developments in information storage, retrieval, and access (Jonsen et al., 2002; Wingfield and Foster, 2002). While computerization of pharmacy and medical records enhances patient care, it can allow ready availability of patient records to third parties such as employers, government agencies, payers, and family members. This increased availability threatens patient and professional control over sensitive information.

HIPAA took effect on April 14, 2003, and is one of the most significant pieces of federal legislation to affect pharmacy practice since the Omnibus Budget Reconciliation Act of 1990 (OBRA) (Spies and Van Dusen, 2003). HIPAA is also considered to be the first comprehensive federal regulation designed to safeguard the privacy and security of PHI. Thus, every pharmacy that conducts certain financial and administrative transactions electronically, such as billing, must be in compliance with its regulations. HIPAA prescribes a framework for the use and disclosure of health information for treatment, payment, and health care operations at all health care institutions, including pharmacies (Giacalone and Cacciatore, 2003; Spies and Van Dusen, 2003). HIPAA was written to "enhance the efficiency and effectiveness of data exchange for administrative and financial transactions while improving the security and privacy of healthcare information" (Mackowiak, 2003).

Confidentiality has always played a key role in pharmacy practice, and the new HIPAA guidelines do not replace state pharmacy statutes and regulations. In fact, HIPAA essentially put into law what pharmacists had been doing on their own for decades. However, HIPAA does provide strict guidelines as to what a pharmacy can do with patient health information. It also provides important rights to patients, such as "the right to access the information, the right to seek details of the disclosure of the information, and the right to view the pharmacy's policies and procedures regarding the confidential information" (Spies and Van Dusen, 2003).

Compliance with HIPAA is mandatory. The Privacy Rule of HIPAA gives pharmacies some flexibility to create their own privacy rules and procedures. "The Privacy Rule requires each pharmacy to take reasonable steps to limit the use or disclosure of, and requests for, PHI defined as individually identifiable health information transmitted or maintained in any form and via any medium" (Spies and Van Dusen, 2003). Examples of PHI include prescriptions and patient record systems. To assure confidentiality of patient information, pharmacies must employ reasonable policies and procedures that limit how PHI is used, disclosed, and requested. Further, pharmacies must post their complete Notice of Privacy Practices within the facility and on their Web site, if one exists.

It has been stated that "although privacy is an important issue, efforts to protect it may conflict with social needs, including the ability of health professionals to exchange information when caring for a patient, the right of parents to sensitive health information concerning their children, and the use of data for research, public health, or audit purposes" (Jonsen et al., 2002). It is the responsibility of the health care provider to become familiar with regulations and policies and be an advocate for better control of information and for improved policies and laws to safeguard it.

THE PRINCIPLE OF FIDELITY

The principle of fidelity, or "faithfulness," relates to the patient–provider relationship. It is based on the principle that health care professionals are expected to be loyal or faithful to their patients. Society has understood that a special type of relationship is created once a patient begins receiving services from his or her health care providers. These are relationships in which both are working together, one as a recipient and one as a "learned professional who is acting ethically." The ethics of medicine have traditionally directed providers to attend exclusively to the needs of their patients and to act in ways that best benefit them. Ethical problems, brought on by multiple responsibilities, can arise when it is unclear which responsibilities have priority or when it appears that duty to one's patient is in conflict with other responsibilities (Jonsen et al., 2002). It is clear, though, that fidelity to patients sometimes requires a subordination of self-interest on the part of the health care provider (Jonsen et al., 2002).

Pharmacists, like all health care providers, do have multiple loyalties—to family, to friends, to a religious faith, to a community, and to other personal, professional, and financial obligations. Thus, pharmacists at times may experience loyalties that pull them in opposing directions and find it difficult to know which choice(s) must be made. For example, pharmacists who promote the use of vitamins or other OTC products to patients who clearly do not need them may be enhancing their financial well-being but are doing so at the expense of their patients, thus violating the ethics of fiduciary responsibility. Pharmacists who refuse to confront physicians about inappropriate prescribing because they want to ensure that physicians will continue to send their patients to a particular pharmacy are also displaying a misplaced sense of professional responsibility and fiduciary ethics. Again, when pharmacists are more attentive to the desires of those signing their paychecks than the health care needs of their patients, they are in a conflict-of-interest situation and in violation of fiduciary responsibility.

Ethically speaking, the pharmacist's main responsibility for having the "privileges and rights of a learned professional" should be the welfare of patients he or she serves. The code of ethics speaks to this when it describes a covenantal relationship between a pharmacist and patient. It would be easy to create a list of dos and don'ts for pharmacists to follow if it were not for the reality that situations encountered within patient–provider relationships are often complex. Thus, the principle of fiduciary responsibility must be considered when working with patients on a case-by-case basis. Patients have the right to be treated with compassion and to receive humane, sensitive care from their providers in a manner that will help them make the best decisions they can. Patients must be able to trust that providers will put the patient's welfare as their primary concern. This is the essence of the "helping" role of the health care professional.

How Can Pharmacists Resolve Ethical Dilemmas?

To best reach ethical decisions, you and your colleagues must use a structured approach for identifying, analyzing, and resolving ethical dilemmas. There are many guides designed to help medical professionals through a decision-making process to reach an ethical decision. One such guide (MacDonald, 1998) offers a simple eight-step approach (see Box 14.2) that provides structure to the decision-making process and considers all relevant aspects of the situation. When faced with an ethical or moral dilemma, you should follow these guidelines in a stepwise progression:

1. Recognize that the decision has moral importance created by conflicts between two or more values or ideals.
2. Identify who the interested parties are, who has a stake in the decision, and what the relationship is between the parties. Consider their relationship with you, each other, and relevant institutions. Ask yourself whether those relationships bring special obligations or unidentified expectations.
3. Consider and identify the values or principles, such as autonomy, honesty, and loyalty, that may be at stake in making the decision.
4. Carefully weigh the benefits and burdens of the case. Benefits may include promotion of health and prevention of suffering and disease, whereas burdens may include causing physical or emotional pain or imposing undue financial burdens.
5. Look for analogous cases in the literature or among colleagues. Can you think of similar decisions you have heard of? What course of action was taken? Ask yourself how the case at hand is similar to that one? How is it different?
6. Consult with colleagues and other relevant advisors. Time permitting and without violating patient confidentiality, discuss your decision with as many persons as have a stake in it. Gather opinions and always remember to ask for reasons behind those opinions.

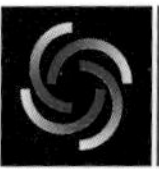

Box 14.2 Eight Steps in an Ethical Decision-Making Process

1. Recognize the moral dimensions.
2. Identify all stakeholders and interested parties.
3. Think through the shared values or principles involved.
4. Weigh the benefits and burdens.
5. Look for analogous cases.
6. Discuss the case with relevant parties and gather opinions.
7. Consider the legal and organizational rules involved.
8. Reflect on how comfortable you are with the decision.

7. Consider the state and/or federal laws involved. Some decisions are, without a doubt, appropriately based on legal considerations. Ethical decisions may also be influenced by rules set by professional organizations, such as the APhA Code of Ethics for Pharmacists. Further, institutions (hospitals, managed care organizations, and others) may have policies that limit available options.
8. Ask yourself whether you are comfortable with the decision. Can you live with the decision? Are there still aspects of the case you have not fully considered? Is your reasoning sound and based on the best interests of the patient?

Analyzing Patient Cases

Three patient cases were described at the beginning of this chapter and are analyzed here according to the ethical principles involved. As you reread each case, before you read the analysis, think about whether you would solve the case any differently now that you have read this chapter.

In Case Study 14.1, it is obvious that Ms. Edwards neither understands the purpose of drug treatment nor the medication's possible side effects. Thus, it could be argued that she has not actually given informed consent to treatment. Arguments against providing information may revolve around fears that Ms. Edwards may not take the medication she needs to treat her medical condition if she is aware of the side effects. The principle invoked in this case is beneficence—doing something that you decide is in her best interest. Other arguments against informing Ms. Edwards may focus on the physician, on the belief that it is the physician's responsibility to inform patients or the physician's right to choose not to provide her with certain information about her treatment. Other arguments may focus on your fears about antagonizing physicians by acting contrary to their wishes and jeopardizing physician referrals to the pharmacy.

The principle of autonomy and the patient's right to determine what will be done to her body argues in favor of providing information about the medication, including its purpose and side effects. You may need to call Ms. Edwards' physician to gather further information pertinent to her treatment or to consult with the physician on how informed consent should take place. Nevertheless, Ms. Edwards has the right to this information and must be informed before she begins taking the medication.

This case highlights the potential conflict of interest facing you in which self-interest or allegiances to others (e.g., physicians) are allowed to override the interests of your patients. The right of the patient to fidelity in the patient–pharmacist relationship is threatened by such a position. You may put yourself in a compromised position to take the physician's position over the patient's needs. Although the principles of beneficence and autonomy may be in conflict in this case, the right of self-determination by the patient is so fundamental as to be paramount. Ms. Edwards has the right to information about her medication, regardless of whether that information would affect her decision to initiate treatment.

Case Study 14.2 involves a decision on whether to reveal confidential information (that James is not taking his antiseizure medication regimen) to other parties. The injunction against release of information without patient consent is strongly held and is based in part on the patient's right of self-determination. It is up to James to decide what information is transmitted to other parties about his medical treatment. The argument for breaking confidentiality in this situation rests on the principle of beneficence (acting in James' best interests by preventing him from injuring himself in an automobile accident). In fact, you may be justified in breaking confidentiality by invoking a duty to protect innocent people (e.g., those potentially injured in future automobile accidents). However, a decision to inform parents and the police would appear to break confidentiality and violate HIPAA. Thus, you would not want to reveal PHI without the patient's consent.

One approach may be to press James to allow you to discuss the situation with his parents so they can participate in this complex process. This motivation would be based on your desire (beneficence) to help James with his treatment. Informing James' physician would generally not be considered a breach of confidentiality, since his physician initiated treatment and since medical information can legitimately be shared with other health professionals involved in a patient's care. Possibly you and James' physician could discuss how to approach James and his parents about this important issue.

When reviewing Megan's case, consider the following questions:

What is the ethical dilemma?
What additional facts may be needed to help you reach a decision?
What alternatives might you consider in resolving this dilemma?
What ethical principles are involved in the decision?
What alternative would you choose and why?
How would you proceed in carrying out your decision?

In listing the ethical principles involved with this case, you probably identified patient confidentiality and beneficence as two of the most important principles.

The first principle implies that, as a pharmacist, you must protect the confidential nature of the patient–provider relationship and therefore must not discuss this issue with Megan's parents. On the other hand, this may conflict with your need to do something to act in Megan's best interest (beneficence). You may feel compelled to tell her parents (since she is a minor) and get them involved in dealing with Megan's medical, psychological, and social issues. It is important to note that those who have not reached the age of 18 are generally considered not to be autonomous; thus, many would argue that it is not unethical for a pharmacist to reveal information to the parents.

In evaluating each approach, the confidentiality issues appear to be clearer than the beneficence issues. Confidentiality simply states that you should not tell Megan's parents without her consent. You may resolve the confidentiality issue by urging Megan to grant you permission to speak with her parents based on your appeal that, in the long run, it will be best for all parties concerned. The beneficence issues are more complex, since you need to identify the real underlying issues. You must ask yourself, "Am I really looking out for Megan's interest or am I responding to my own parental instincts?" In addition, you may be responding out of fear of what would happen if Megan's parents eventually found out that you knew about her situation. Fear of losing friends and their business should not be the primary motivators in this situation. You and your colleagues may certainly break confidentiality when a patient's life is in danger, such as when concerns about suicide exist or there is an imminent threat of bodily harm. However, resolving a confidentiality issue when the threat to a patient's health is more psychological than physical is more difficult.

Contemporary Topics in Pharmacy Care

This chapter concludes with a discussion of a contemporary issue that seems to affect many pharmacists. It is presented as a means of summarizing several key factors in ethical decision making.

CONSCIENTIOUS OBJECTION

Discuss with a few colleagues your response to the following scenario BEFORE reading the discussion that follows it:

Do pharmacists have the right to refuse to dispense a drug when presented with a valid prescription that they know is to be used in a treatment that is in conflict with their personal beliefs? What duty do pharmacists have to the patient in this situation?

Discussion

Advancements in the production, availability, and distribution of medication, as well as changes in societal beliefs, have placed pharmacists at the forefront of a number of ethical and moral dilemmas. Pharmacists form a critical link in the chain of drug distribution to the patient by dispensing drugs that are only available by prescription. In essence, they are the "gatekeepers" who determine whether dispensing a prescription order serves a legitimate medical purpose (Joranson and Gilson, 2001). It is clearly written in state pharmacy laws that it is the pharmacist's duty to refuse to dispense if, in the pharmacist's professional judgment, the prescription does not seem valid or could cause harm to the patient. But what are the ethical issues surrounding pharmacists' ability to conscientiously object to dispensing a medication? What happens when a pharmacist's ethical, moral, or religious beliefs conflict with the patient's beliefs and medical needs?

CONSCIENTIOUS OBJECTION REVISITED

Conscientious objection raises important issues and questions relating to individual rights and public health. Cantor and Baum (2004) ask, "Who prevails when the needs of the patient and the morals of the provider collide?" Many arguments can be made for and against a pharmacist's right to object. Cantor and Baum (2004) argue that pharmacists should exercise independent judgment because, like other health care professionals, they have the credentials and experience needed to exhibit sound judgment and to be an integral member of the health care team and "thus, it seems inappropriate and condescending to question a pharmacist's right to exercise personal judgment." Further, proponents of conscientious objection reflect that professionals should not have to forsake their morals as a condition of employment. For instance, "ethics and law allow physicians, nurses, and physician assistants to refuse to participate in abortions and other reproductive services" and therefore, pharmacists should be afforded the same respect.

Opponents of conscientious objection argue that once pharmacists choose to enter the profession, they are bound by certain fiduciary duties, and therefore, they are supposed to place the patient's interests before their own immediate interests (Cantor and Baum, 2004). Further, they argue that certain principles in the pharmacist's Code of Ethics weigh against conscientious objection. Specifically, "a pharmacist respects the autonomy and dignity of each patient" and "a pharmacist serves individual, community, and societal needs" (APhA, 1994). Finally, opponents reflect that refusal to dispense has great potential for abuse and discrimination because pharmacists are privy to personal and sensitive patient information and could refuse to fill a prescription if they mistakenly make judgments relating to people's behaviors (Cantor and Baum, 2004). For example, pharmacists may refuse to fill a prescription for the treatment of HIV on the basis that some HIV-positive individuals may engage in what the pharmacist believes to be immoral behavior. According to Cantor and Baum (2004), "such objections go beyond conscience to become invasive."

At its annual meeting in 1998, the APhA adopted a conscience clause that addresses conscientious objection, stating, "APhA recognizes the individual pharmacist's right to exercise conscientious refusal and supports the establishment of systems to ensure patient access to legally prescribed therapy without compromising the pharmacist's right to conscientious refusal" (APhA, 1998). Prior to 1998, no state had adopted a conscience clause, "a declaration of conscientious objection to an issue…which specifically addresses pharmacist liability should the decision be made to refuse to dispense a prescription" (Harvey et al., 2006). Since then, many states have adopted legislation that offers some level of legal protection for health care professionals who refuse to provide certain reproductive services. As of July 2010, 46 states have passed legislation explicitly allowing health care professionals and some institutions to refuse to provide or participate in abortion, contraceptive, or sterilization services due to religious or moral objections. Laws in five states (Arkansas, Georgia, Idaho, Mississippi, and South Dakota) explicitly permit pharmacists to refuse to provide contraceptives on moral or religious grounds and protect them from liability because of their refusal, while in Arizona, the law states it is the pharmacist's duty to fill all valid prescriptions. By contrast, seven states (Alabama, California, Hawaii, Massachusetts, New Hampshire, Vermont, and Washington) have given permission to pharmacists to fill emergency contraceptives if there is a "collaborative practice agreement" with a physician or, as is done in three states (California, Maine, and New Mexico), the state has allowed emergency contraception to be dispended under "state protocol" (Guttmacher Institute, 2010).

Case Study 14.4 reveals the ethical issues surrounding conscientious objection. This case involves the ethical principles of patient autonomy, provider fidelity, and nonmalfeasance. Patients expect their health care providers, including pharmacists, to use their professional judgment to make sound decisions that are factual and objective and not based on personal judgments. Patients reveal sensitive and personal information to their pharmacist, and for that trust they expect a certain degree of loyalty. Moral dilemmas arise when the pharmacist feels morally unable to honor the fiduciary relationship with the patient by filling a valid prescription. By not filling the prescription, the pharmacist may be seen as assuming a paternalistic role, "knowing what is best for that patient," thus compromising patient autonomy. It is important to understand that the trend in health care is toward empowering patients to control their own health care, and autonomy is best expressed by a freedom to choose based on informed decision-making.

Pharmacists who choose not to fill a valid prescription for a drug that is to be used in a treatment that is in conflict with personal beliefs must be informed of state legislation regarding conscientious objection and their employers' stand on the topic. Pharmacists have a duty to provide access to drugs to people who need them, and patients are entitled to the treatment initiated by the physician. Thus, alternate arrangements need to be made to help the patient. For instance, the pharmacist may have another pharmacist fill the prescription, refer to another pharmacy, or, at a minimum, contact the prescribing physician.

Pharmacists need to be aware of the implications of conscientious objection not only to the patient but also to their employer and coworkers. According to Harvey et al. (2006), "when a pharmacist takes a job, that employee is obligated to comply with the employer's policies and procedures... when such personal and volatile issues occur without notice in the workplace, people are caught off guard." Thus, it is preferable that pharmacists explore these sensitive topics with employers in an open discussion before hiring, thus avoiding potentially volatile situations that are not conducive to customer satisfaction or patient welfare.

A second example of conscientious objection involves filling prescriptions for assisted-suicide situations. In 1997 physician-assisted suicide became a legal option for terminally ill patients in Oregon. The Death with Dignity Act allows physicians to write prescriptions for lethal doses of medications (Oregon Department of Human Services, 2005). Similar to the issue of emergency contraception, the dispensing of life-ending drugs presents ethical dilemmas for pharmacists. Some pharmacists feel that it is their right to know when a prescription will be used for a life-ending event.

To help guide pharmacists through the decision-making process in assisted suicide, the ASHP in 1999 issued the "ASHP Statement on Pharmacists Decision-Making in Assisted Suicide." In this document, ASHP reinforces that "the basic tenet of the profession is to provide care and affirm life." Further, the ASHP (1999) reflected that the patient-provider relationship is based on trust, respect for patient autonomy, confidentiality, and decision making, and it is the pharmacist's duty to ensure that the patient and the health care team are informed of all pharmacotherapeutic options available in treating the patient's condition. It also states that the patient has the right to determine his or her own therapeutic option, including end-of-life decisions. Pharmacists must respect the patient's decision and maintain confidentiality "regardless of whether they agree with the values underlying the patient's choice of treatment or decision to forgo any particular treatment" (ASHP, 1999). Finally, ASHP also supported conscientious objection by stating "pharmacists must retain their rights to participate or not in morally, religiously, or ethically troubling therapies." Thus, pharmacists are left to consider not only the state regulations concerning assisted suicide and conscientious objection, but also the ethical and moral principles involved in the patient–provider relationship.

Summary

As a pharmacist, you must understand the ethical principles of nonmalfeasance, beneficence, autonomy, honesty and truth-telling, informed consent, confidentiality, and fidelity that serve as foundations for ethical decision making in health care (see Box 14.3). The obligation to respect patient autonomy, protect confidentiality of patient information, serve patient welfare, and treat patients with respect and compassion are fundamental duties for any health care professional. Using a systematic decision-making process when ethical dilemmas arise and principles seem to compete can help you and your colleagues reach decisions that are ethically valid.

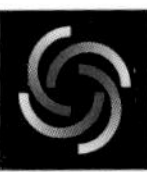

Box 14.3 Quick Guide to a Systematic Approach to Competing Ethical Principles in Pharmacy Practice

PRINCIPLE OF NONMALFEASANCE

a) You should not do something that will cause harm.
b) Ask yourself: "Is what I am about to do likely to help the patient or harm the patient?"

PRINCIPLE OF BENEFICENCE

a) Are you doing what is right and for the better "good" of the patient?
b) Your main concern is patient welfare and not your own self-interests.
c) Ask yourself, "Is what I am about to do likely to be medically helpful?"

PRINCIPLE OF AUTONOMY

a) You accept that a patient has the inherent right of self-determination, the right to refuse to take medications, and the right to be educated on the pros and cons of his or her medication.
b) Your main concern is the patient's capacity to deal with the complexity of any drug and its regimen or its side effects. Surrogate decision making may be used when a patient's wishes are unclear or unknown, or if a surrogate is used in a cultural capacity.
c) You ask, "Is this patient capable of understanding or acting on the advice I am giving and is the request for my services going beyond what is considered good MTM?"

PRINCIPLE OF HONESTY AND TRUTH-TELLING

a) You have a duty to tell the truth and be honest.
b) You should not let technical jargon about medications obscure truth and fact.
c) You ask, "Is what I am saying an honest attempt at communicating information in a manner understood by lay people?"

PRINCIPLE OF INFORMED CONSENT

a) You have a duty to inform patients of the pros and cons of their medications.
b) You have a responsibility to assure the public that their knowledge is current and verifiable.
c) You ask, "Is the information that I am providing going to help the patient make an informed decision?"

PRINCIPLE OF CONFIDENTIALITY

a) You have a covenant with patients that complete and absolute confidentiality will underlie any relationship.
b) You must comply with professional laws and regulations, which vary across federal and state lines, regarding disclosure of health information to public health authorities and third party organizations.

(Continued)

Box 14.3 cont.

c) You ask, "Is what I am communicating to a colleague or another individual likely to cause an issue should someone other than the patient act on this information?"

PRINCIPLE OF FIDELITY

a) You have a duty not to abandon a patient once a relationship has been established.
b) You may voluntarily terminate relationships with patients when you feel uncomfortable filling their prescription if you give them a reasonable amount of time to make other arrangements and give help with making alternative arrangements.
c) You ask, "Is there a conflict between me and this patient that cannot be resolved by third party arbitration, ethics committee, or professional group, and if I go forward on my own, could I be construed as abandoning a patient in need?"

REVIEW QUESTIONS

1. **Describe "beneficence" and compare it with "fidelity."**
2. **Compare and contrast the principles of autonomy and paternalism in the patient–provider relationship.**
3. **State some of the limitations of "informed consent."**
4. **Describe HIPAA as it relates to confidentiality.**
5. **Describe a process for pharmacists to use in resolving ethical dilemmas.**

REFERENCES

Accreditation Council for Pharmacy Education, 2007. Retrieved July 2010 from http://www.acpe-accredit.org.

American Pharmaceutical Association. APhA Code of Ethics, adopted by the membership on October 27, 1994.

American Pharmaceutical Association. Current APhA statements related to the practice environment and quality of work life issues. Pharmacists Conscience Clause, *Journal of the American Pharmaceutical Association* 38:417, 1998.

American Society of Health-System Pharmacists. ASHP Statement on Pharmacists Decision-Making on Assisted Suicide. *American Journal of Health-System Pharmacy* 56:1661–1664, 1999.

Beauchamp T. Informed consent. In Veatch RM (ed.). *Medical Ethics*. Boston, MA: Jones and Bartlett, 1989.

Cady, R. Informed consent for adult patients: A review of basic principles. *American Journal of Maternal and Child Nursing* 25:106–108, 2000.

Cantor J, Baum K. The limits of conscientious objection—may pharmacists refuse to fill prescriptions for emergency contraception? *New England Journal of Medicine* 351:2008–2012, 2004.

Curlin FA, Lawrence RE, Chin MH, et al. Religion, conscience, and controversial clinical practices, *New England Journal of Medicine* 357:593–600, 2007.

Da Silva CHM, Cunha RLG, Tonaco RB, et al. Not telling the truth in the patient-physician relationship. *Bioethics* 17:417–424, 2003.

Dhillon S, Duggan C, Joshua AE. What part should pharmacists play in providing medicines-related information? *The Pharmaceutical Journal* 266:364–366, 2001.

Gallup Poll. 2009. Retrieved July 2010 from http:www.gallup.com/poll103123/lobbyists-debut-bottom-honesty-ethics-list.aspx.

Giacalone RP, Cacciatore GG. HIPAA and its impact on pharmacy practice. *American Journal of Health System Pharmacy* 60:433–445, 2003.

Guttmacher Institute. State Policies in Brief: Refusing to Provide Health Services. New York, NY, July 2010. Retrieved July 2010 from http://www.guttmacher.org/statecenter/spibs/spib_RPHS.pdf.

Harvey SE, Lu E, Rivas O, Rodgers DA. Do pharmacists have the right to refuse to dispense a prescription based on personal beliefs? 2006. Retrieved October 12, 2010 from http://www.nm-pharmacy.com/body_rights.htm.

Institute of Medicine. *Crossing the Quality Chasm: A New Health System for the 21st Century*. Institute of Medicine of the National Academies. Washington, DC, 2001.

Institute for Safe Medication Practices. *Protecting U.S. Citizens from Inappropriate Medication Use*. Institute for Safe Medication Practices. Huntingdon Valley, PA, 2007.

Jonsen AR, Siegler M, Winslade WJ. *Clinical Ethics: A Practical Approach to Ethical Decisions in Clinical Medicine*. New York, NY: McGraw-Hill, 2002.

Joranson DE, Gilson AM. Pharmacists' knowledge of and attitudes toward opioid pain medications in relation to federal and state policies. *Journal of the American Pharmaceutical Association* 41:213–220, 2001.

MacDonald C. A guide to moral decision making. In *Everyday Ethics: Putting the Code into Practice*. Toronto: Canadian Nurses Association, 1998.

Mackowiak LR. Pharmacists and HIPAA. *American Journal of Health System Pharmacy* 60:431–432, 2003.

Munson R. *Intervention and Reflection: Basic Issues in Medical Ethics*. Belmont, CA: Wadsworth/Thomson Learning, 2000.

Oregon Department of Human Services. *Seventh Annual Report on Oregon's Death with Dignity Act*. March 10, 2005.

Quallich SA. The practice of informed consent. *Dermatology Nursing* 17:49–51, 2005.

Spies AR, Van Dusen V. HIPAA: Practical application of the federal patient privacy act. *U.S. Pharmacist* 28, 2003. Retrieved August 21, 2006 from http://www.uspharmacist.com.

Tindall WN, Millonig MK. *Pharmaceutical Care: Insights from Community Pharmacists*. Boca Raton, FL: CRC Press, 2003.

Veatch RM. *The Basics of Bioethics*. Upper Saddle River, NJ: Prentice Hall, 2000.

Virginia Commonwealth University School of Pharmacy. Curriculum Goals for the Doctor of Pharmacy Program, 2010. Retrieved July 2010 from http://www.pharmacy.vcu.edu.

Wingfield J. Consent and decision making for patients who lack capacity: What should pharmacists know? *The Pharmaceutical Journal* 271:463–464, 2003.

Wingfield J, Foster C. Consent and confidentiality: Legal implications of electronic transmissions of prescriptions. *The Pharmaceutical Journal* 269:328–331, 2002.

Zellmer WA. *Role of Pharmacy Organizations in Transforming the Profession*. APhA Annual Meeting, March 2001, San Francisco, CA.

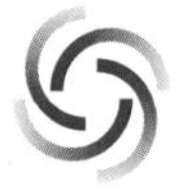

Index

Page numbers followed by f denote figures; page numbers followed by b denote boxed information.

A

B

C

D

E

J

K

L

M

N

O

P

R